Remember When

My life with Alzheimer's

Fiona Phillips

MACMILLAN

First published 2025 by Macmillan
an imprint of Pan Macmillan
The Smithson, 6 Briset Street, London EC1M 5NR
EU representative: Macmillan Publishers Ireland Ltd, 1st Floor,
The Liffey Trust Centre, 117–126 Sheriff Street Upper,
Dublin 1 D01 YC43
Associated companies throughout the world

ISBN 978-1-0350-7487-7

1 3 5 7 9 8 6 4 2

A CIP catalogue record for this book is available from the British Library.

Typeset in Adobe Caslon Pro by Palimpsest Book Production Ltd, Falkirk, Stirlingshire
Printed and bound in the UK using 100% Renewable Electricity by CPI Group (UK) Ltd

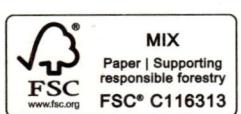

Visit **www.panmacmillan.com** to read more about all our books
and to buy them.

Remember When

To Martin, Nat and Mackenzie – the men I love.

I don't dedicate to you the story of loss that this book tells.
Instead, I dedicate the good times and laughter we have shared.

Treasure those memories for me.

Foreword

Fiona

Autumn 2023

In front of me, on the glossy white kitchen table of our family home lies a huge pile of old magazine and newspaper cuttings. They are interviews with me over the past forty years of my life as a television presenter and journalist. There's a picture of me in a very nineties red power suit with my *GMTV* breakfast show co-host Eamonn Holmes's arm draped around me (who thought that was a good pose?!). And there are some hilarious snaps of me, all hot and sweaty, when I appeared with Brendan Cole as my partner (for a few weeks, at least) on the BBC's *Strictly Come Dancing*. Then there are the neatly snipped-out and filed pages of the *Daily Mirror*, where my weekly opinion column appeared each Saturday.

On the whitewashed shelf along the kitchen wall, between a spider plant and a pomegranate-scented candle, are framed pictures of my family. There's me and my husband, Martin, smiling outside a film premiere. And another of the pair of us with our gorgeous boys, Nathaniel and Mackenzie, when they were little on the beach in Dorset, where we used to go on holiday.

I look up through the kitchen windows, out to the shady patch of grass surrounding our south London home, where the boys used to play football hour after hour after hour until every last blade of green had been trampled to mud.

Everywhere I look there are memories. I know they are there. They must be there . . . That's what a home is – a house built from memories.

And yet so many of them feel out of my reach now.

It's like I stretch out to touch them, to recall the photo shoots I see in the magazines or the moment we took that photograph on the beach by the windbreaks in Dorset, but then just as I'm about to grasp it, the memory skips away from me. And I can't catch up with it. Like trying to chase a £5 note that's fallen out of your purse on a gusty day. Each time I think I've caught it, it whips away again and then I'm left frustrated and confused. Or imagine having a nightmare where it's pitch-black and you are desperately searching for someone you love in a house you've never visited before. I feel like I'm wandering from room to room in that house, looking for the person, then when I finally think I've found the right room, I start scrabbling in my handbag for the door key. There's so much stuff in my bag that it takes me ages to lay my hand on the key, but eventually I can feel it, pull it out and try to fit it in the lock. I push it in one way and then another. Finally, it clicks in place and I turn it. I gently push the door open, but then, in that very moment, I sense the person I love has disappeared again.

They're gone. The memory has gone. And I'm all alone.

And that's how it is for me now, living with Alzheimer's.

That's what 'they' (whoever 'they' are) call it: 'living with Alzheimer's'. Not that there's any choice. It's not like living with ugly curtains or living with noisy neighbours. You can rip down curtains or move away from a rowdy house next door, but I'm not able to escape Alzheimer's. It's staying right here with me.

I'd just turned sixty when I was diagnosed with the disease in early 2022, although it was probably stalking me long before that. I feel now like Alzheimer's had been coming my way, secretly, stealthily creeping into my brain, for years. Who knows? Maybe it was within me somewhere since the day I was born, just waiting for the moment to explode in all its awfulness.

There are few families anywhere in this country who haven't been impacted by this terrible illness in some way, be they parents, partners or children. Certainly, my family has had more than its fair share of it.

Alzheimer's has been in my life for almost as long as I can remember. That really isn't meant to be a joke, so maybe instead I should just say it's always been there. My grandma, Mum, Dad, my Uncle Barry . . . They were all taken by it. It's like a curse that keeps coming back to claim us.

For those of you fortunate enough not to have been touched by this disease, let me give you a brief explanation. Alzheimer's disease is the most common form of dementia and it affects people's ability to remember things, their behaviour and their ability to think. Generally, it starts with feeling a bit confused and then little by little, day by day, it becomes harder and harder to remember things or to function in a normal way.

It's caused by a build-up of plaque (like you get on your teeth if you don't brush them) around cells in the brain. After a while the brain cells are destroyed or die and then, well, you can imagine what happens then. But if you're thinking, *Hang on, this is an old person's disease*, well, you're quite right. There's about a million people in the UK with dementia at the moment, according to research by the Alzheimer's Society. Just 70,000 of them are under sixty-five and are described as having 'early-onset' dementia so I'm part of a pretty exclusive set! Although it's a set I'd have done anything to avoid.

In this book I hope to explain how month by month, Alzheimer's has changed my life. I say that 'I hope' because as I begin now, I cannot be certain whether I will be able to finish the book myself or whether the confusion that seems to be growing thicker all the time will block me before I can tell you all that I want to say.

And there's so much I want to say. About all the wonderful times I've had, my kind, brave sons, the tremendous fun I had on TV, about meeting Martin – the man I love, the love of my life – and all he has done for me over the past couple of years.

I hope this book can show people a little about what it's like to live with Alzheimer's, how frightening and confusing it is, but also how much of life can still bring joy and a feeling of being valued. I used to hear so many people say, 'Well, if I get Alzheimer's, take me in the corner and shoot me.' But I don't want to be shot. I want to go for dinner with my husband to a quiet restaurant or walk through the park when the autumn leaves are coming down from the trees. I want to watch Chelsea beat Arsenal 3–0 at home. I want our son Nat to come home on leave from the army and give me one of his bear-like hugs. I want our youngest son Mackenzie to bring me a cup of tea and a biscuit when we sit watching TV together.

I want to be *me*.

I'm not going to be sugar-coating anything in this book – this is a shit situation that I'm in and I've just got to deal with it. Apologies if my language isn't very 'Breakfast TV' but my life isn't very 'Breakfast TV' these days either. And it happens to so many people. So many families are having to cope with the fear and confusion that comes when the illness sweeps in, changing everything. Which is why, more than anything, I want this book to encourage everyone to treasure the memories they have, as well as the ones they are yet to make, because you never know when these may be taken away from you. Memory is such a huge part of what defines us as people and when it starts to ebb away, much of what we are goes with it.

Above all, I want to plead, demand, beg that the work and funding into research that will prevent others from being hit by this disease continues. It's good to know how much progress is going on scientifically that might slow, or even one day stop altogether, the progress of Alzheimer's for future sufferers but, I'll be honest, it bloody hurts too, knowing most likely that it will be too late for me.

Here, I also need to be honest about the extent of my illness for those of you reading this book. You might be thinking, *Well, she can't be that bad if she's sitting down and typing a 300-or-so-page book*. The reality is I couldn't be writing this at all without my husband Martin and my closest friends, who are nudging me to remember moments of my life that I have forgotten. And they are helping me articulate more clearly the thoughts I once had that are now harder for me to reach. I used to be able to talk to anyone about anything (a skill inherited from my mum) and then I made a career out of chatting to people on television. Nowadays, I can find talking about my life agonizingly difficult. Sometimes I get halfway through a sentence and I can't remember where I was heading with it or the word I was looking for. It feels awful.

A lot of people these days have ghostwriters to help shape their memories and thoughts into a story that makes sense. Usually, it's all a big secret and the readers are led to believe that some great *Love Island* star or teen pop sensation has just knocked out 90,000 words in their spare time. I could have done the same, but that wouldn't have been honest, so I want you to know that a ghostwriter, Alison Phillips, is helping me put together the memories I do have for this story. Alison and I have known each other for more than twenty years, since I started writing a weekly column at the *Mirror*, where she worked. In the old days, we would enjoy long, gossipy lunches together and, more recently, we've been going for walks around Clapham Common as I try to make sense of this illness. I know if there comes a point when I can't continue with this book, she will work with Martin to make sure it tells my story honestly – the way it has to be told.

Events from years ago are easier for me. Maybe that's because they've been lodged in my head for longer and so they're stuck there more firmly. It's the recent stuff that seems to shift around my mind, refusing to stay still.

Alzheimer's disease gets progressively worse, so I have to be aware that as I write this story over the next year or so, my memory will probably deteriorate. I've given everyone strict instructions that no matter how things progress, I want to keep on trying to give an honest account of how I'm feeling. I want it to be in my own words and, if my own words don't always make sense, that's just how it is. No point in tidying up my words to give a false impression of how I am!

During all those years sitting on the sofa presenting *GMTV*, the thing I tried to do above all else was be honest with my viewers. And I'm not going to stop being honest with people now, even if things become a bit messy. If it does all start to get really messy . . . well, that's where Martin steps in. Hopefully he'll explain the bits that I can't. It's he who has got me through all this and continues to do so each day. Hopefully he'll help you get to the end of this book without giving up too!

If you or someone you love is in the early stages of Alzheimer's, please don't compare what you can write or say or remember with what I've put together in this book – there has been a lot of help! I just hope it brings you some comfort.

Twenty years ago, I looked after my lovely mum when she had everything stripped away from her by Alzheimer's. And then I did it again when my dad also fell into its clutches (I'll tell you all about this as this book goes on). I can still remember how tough it was to care for someone with this illness and how utterly bloody terrifying it is when you get the diagnosis yourself. In both situations, maybe the very worst thing was that aching sense of being completely alone, even when I was surrounded by people I loved and who loved me. The nature of this illness is that it isolates its sufferers. So, if this book achieves one thing, it's that I want you to know that you are not alone. There are hundreds of thousands of us dealing with this illness, and together we are not alone.

Remember: you are not alone.

Foreword

Martin

Autumn 2023

As Fiona starts work on this book, towards the end of 2023, I really hope you won't be hearing too much from me! This is Fiona's story to tell. She is the one who has worked so hard to support her parents through their battles with Alzheimer's and now, in some supreme act of cruelty, she is having to face the same challenge herself.

Fiona and I met back in 1995, when we were both working for the breakfast show *GMTV*. We'd known each other vaguely earlier than that, but it was in 1995, when she was the show's Los Angeles correspondent, that we became a couple.

There are many things I loved and admired then – and now – about the woman who became my wife, but one of them was that she was a truly great journalist. More than most, Fiona understands the importance of telling difficult stories to a huge audience in the hope it might do some good. When her parents were both ill in the early 2000s, she frequently wrote about Alzheimer's disease – the struggles to get early diagnosis, the lack of support for loved ones and the slowness in finding treatments compared to research into other diseases. Fiona believed that by shining a light on the way Alzheimer's is regarded, she could help sufferers and their families in the future. Now with this book, once again she is determined to use her experiences to bring comfort to others and to help answer the questions with which sufferers are faced when they get this terrible diagnosis. And let me tell you, if Fiona is determined to do something, she does it. Never in my life have I met someone more determined – or, as I more usually describe it, stubborn.

Until the past couple of years, nothing ever stopped Fiona from doing what she wanted when she wanted. Not my best attempts at persuasion, encouragement or even the occasional shouting match could make a difference. But Alzheimer's has changed all that, along with so much else. And so, despite Fiona's determination to complete this story of her life, I know there are parts that are now lost to her, which is why she has asked me to fill in some of the gaps in her memory for this book.

The nature of this illness as it progresses means that those suffering with it are sometimes unable to see situations in the way that people around them do, so I will try to give you the perspective of Fiona's friends and family and show what it's been like for us – her family – watching things change. At first there was our confusion, irritation and a sense of hurt as her behaviour towards us changed over many months. Then came the shock, anger and devastation after her diagnosis in 2022.

Writing this is strange, and I'll be honest, a little uncomfortable for me. I am more used to being 'behind the scenes' than sharing my own thoughts and emotions in public. For almost a decade – since July 2015 – I've been the editor of ITV's *This Morning*, so if you've ever sat down to watch Cat Deeley and Ben Shephard in the mornings, then somewhere behind the scenes will have been me. My job is to constantly come up with a stream of ideas to keep the show fresh and interesting. Over the years we've had our fair share of dramas, some of which I'm sure you'll have seen, but until now I've always liked to stay firmly in the background. Just as I've tried to stay in the background while supporting Fiona.

I never really wanted Fiona and me to become the poster girl and boy for Alzheimer's disease. Despite us both working within showbusiness, we have led a very private life as a family and have always regarded ourselves first and foremost as journalists who report on the news, rather than people who are actually *in* the news themselves. But we understand that Fiona has a public profile and the outpouring of support since she first shared her diagnosis has been incredible. That's why she's writing this now. When we're out for a coffee, people will come up to say hi and ask Fiona how she's getting on. So many people want to talk about how this illness has touched their family. I think it can be so traumatic for them that they just want to share their story with her.

When we went on holiday to Italy soon after Fiona shared her diagnosis publicly, I was a bit anxious about how she would cope on the flight, surrounded by so many people she didn't know. But the crew were so kind and took so much care of her, bringing her water and guiding her to the toilet, even inviting us up to the flight deck to meet the captain. I didn't need to tell them about Fiona's diagnosis – I'm sure they must have read about it in the newspapers – and that took so much stress out of the situation. Over the past couple of years we have both felt incredibly supported by the public.

We know our family's experience is shared by hundreds of thousands across the UK. Seeing the person you love slowly slip away is agonizing, exhausting and often frustrating. Fiona and I have no magic solutions for how to deal with this car crash of emotions – because there aren't any. Our only hope is that the scientists looking for treatments for this truly awful disease will be successful soon and the suffering can be ended. And our enormous pride is in Fiona for her innate determination (OK, stubbornness!) that means her story *will* be told.

1

Fiona

June 2018

I strode out across Clapham Common with the mission of
making it all around the edge and back home again before
Martin got in from work. How I loved the common, with its
expanse of heath, dotted with woodland like a piece of countryside picked up and dropped onto the streets of south-west
London.

It's a stone's throw from our home and even when it's full of
young mums pushing buggies, joggers and skateboarders or
teenagers playing football, there's still space enough to be alone.
To get your head straight, away from the noise and commotion
of the city.

How many years have I been going there? I remember taking
Mackenzie in his pram around and around when he wouldn't
sleep and pushing Nat on the swings in the children's playground. It's incredible to think that they are both grown men:
that summer, Nat had turned twenty and even my baby
Mackenzie was sixteen.

As the boys got older and I wasn't constantly rushing from pillar to post after them while trying to balance childcare with my TV work, I'd wander down to the common for peace, quiet and the sense of freedom it gave me.

That day, the grass was already turning brown after a few weeks of dry weather. A group of kids in school uniforms were sprawled out, enjoying the warmth and a bag of Greggs donuts. A young mum, still with the energy and enthusiasm to bother in the heat, was chasing her giggling toddler around in circles. All about me there was a sense of relaxed summer chill, that sort of 'shoes off, grass beneath your feet, laughing in the sunshine, nothing really matters' feeling.

Well, that's what I saw, but it wasn't what I felt.

It was like looking through a double-glazed window onto another world of which I had no part. It was a strange sense of disconnection. Of seeing others laughing, enjoying the moment, while increasingly I felt, well, nothing. Just flat. Utterly flat.

I hadn't felt completely myself for years. So much of the time there seemed to be a lingering sense of anxiety within me. It was hard to explain to people what the problem was or what had caused it. I just felt uneasy, different and the thought of going places I didn't know or meeting people who were new filled me with dread.

I'd always been very independent and enjoyed my own company, but this was different. That day was particularly bad. I'd hoped that a brisk walk and some fresh air might help. Sometimes it did. But nothing seemed to totally shift this weird sense of unease that had lodged somewhere just below my chest.

It's hard to explain anxiety to someone who has never experienced it, but imagine the kind of sick feeling you might have before an exam or a job interview – and that's just the beginning. Of course what's so odd is there is no exam or job interview, no real reason to feel like this at all. It's like all my nerves are constantly screeching; I'm on high alert as if something really bad is about to happen, like that feeling you get if you hear a crash in another room when you're home alone and you're terrified someone has broken in. But in reality there is nothing to be worried about.

That summer's afternoon I was a fifty-seven-year-old woman with a great husband, whom I loved, and two amazing sons. I lived in a beautiful house and, despite my age, I was still getting regular offers of TV work and writing a weekly column in a national newspaper. But, for the first time in my life, I wasn't snapping up all of those offers. If anything, I avoided having to go anywhere I'd not been before or meeting people I didn't know. Even at home with Martin and the boys, I knew I'd lost my sparkle. I just didn't feel 'up for it' in the same way I used to, though that's not to suggest that before summer 2018 I was always out painting the town red. With Martin and I both spending our careers working in television, we were often invited to nice restaurants or glitzy awards ceremonies, but that had never really been our bag – we'd rather have a few drinks in the local pub or a quiet dinner at home. We worked in showbiz worlds, but our home life had always been very ordinary and settled. Or at least it had been until the anxiety set in and I found even the thought of going out for dinner a bit overwhelming.

You've just got to pull yourself together, Fiona, I told myself that day as I walked around the common. I realize that is a terribly unfashionable thing to say nowadays and we are all encouraged to talk about how we are feeling, but I couldn't really explain how I felt. And I wasn't brought up that way either.

My mum loved me and my two brothers, David and Andrew, to bits, but we weren't spoiled and we certainly weren't encouraged to make a fuss. 'Stop making a spectacle of yourself,' she would have said. 'Just get your coat on and put on your best face for the world.'

Looking back to my childhood – particularly my teens – I can now see how Mum suffered from years of depression and anxiety herself, but she never talked about it and neither did we. None of us ever discussed it. We thought it must be 'her nerves', whatever that was supposed to mean. It was something people used to say in those days. So we just watched silently, horrified and awkward, as she gradually shrank into herself and would quietly cry in her bedroom during 'one of her turns'.

Maybe that sounds strange to people now, but it was entirely normal in the 1970s. It might have been all about free love and free feelings on the West Coast of America, but in the suburbs of Southampton it was, 'Keep the noise down – your mum's got one of her headaches.'

That sunny day in 2018, I was probably feeling similar to the way Mum often felt when she went to lie down in her bedroom. At the time, though, that didn't occur to me, but there was no doubt my sense of anxiety was getting worse.

The previous morning, my agent, Jan, had called me out of the blue. We had worked together for more than a decade and she was responsible for sorting out contracts and deals for any work requests that came in for me. I didn't use an agent in the way that lots of television presenters do to find them work on TV shows or events because most of the time I was able to find my own work. Still, Jan often called with opportunities or suggestions for shows she could put me up for. By then it had reached the point where each time I saw Jan's name pop up on the screen of my mobile phone, I instantly hit the red button to reject the call. It wasn't that I didn't want to speak to her – I loved our chats and having a good old gossip about who was 'in' and who was 'out' in the TV world – but I felt sick at the mere thought of how I was going to come up with another excuse as to why I couldn't do whatever job I'd been offered now.

This time I had plucked up all my courage and accepted the call.

'Hi, Jan, how are you?' I trilled in my very best 'on air' voice.

'I'm great – but how about you? I've got about three different offers for you here . . . A TV ad, a new consumer investigation series and some promotional work. Take your pick!'

'Ha,' I laughed weakly. 'That all sounds . . . well . . . great. Yes, I'd love to do it . . . all of it . . . But I'm just getting on the tube and I can't really talk – can I ring you back?'

Quickly turning the phone off, I stuffed it to the bottom of my handbag. My hands had gone all clammy and my heart was racing at a million miles an hour.

Of course I wasn't on the tube. Or anywhere near it. And of course the reality was there was no way I would be ringing Jan back. I just couldn't do what she was asking – I couldn't work at all. I wanted to so much, but the thought of meeting a whole crew of strangers, having to turn on the old performance for them all . . . It made me feel sick. Physically sick, like I could throw up right there and then.

At the same time, I felt so guilty. Of course I should be working. So why couldn't I just ring Jan back and say, 'Yes, great, sign me up'? She must have been wondering too. But I didn't know the answer and that was what was so truly terrifying.

But the most terrifying thing of all that kept going over and over in my mind like a nightmarish advertising jingle was 'What if you never work again?'

When Martin got in from work that evening, I tried to explain to him how I was feeling. Once again, he suggested we go out for dinner at the weekend to talk it through. Again, I couldn't face it.

'I just feel so, so . . . eurgh,' I said.

'I know,' he said, 'but you might enjoy it when we get there.'

'I won't,' I snapped back. 'I can't face it. You don't understand. I haven't worked now for nearly a year and the longer it goes on, the more I can't cope with the idea of trying anything new. There's nothing wrong with the work I'm being offered, I just don't want to do it.'

'Maybe you need a bit of career time out while you think what you'd really love to do next,' said Martin, ever the TV professional. He was used to dealing with high-maintenance showbiz personalities!

But that annoyed me even more. Because I absolutely was not one of those people and I didn't particularly want his good advice either – all I wanted was to go back to being me.

'It might be time for a change of direction,' he went on. 'You just need some space to work out what that direction should be.'

'It's more than that,' I attempted to argue. 'I feel as though I've lost my oomph – and what if that oomph has upped and left for ever?' I tried laughing to hide what was actually becoming my greatest fear: what if this feeling was permanent?

'I'm sure that's not the case, Fiona,' Martin replied calmly. 'Everyone goes through phases of feeling down and it will come back – I've never met anyone with such energy and such an incredible work ethic as you. But if you're feeling like this, why don't you go to the doctor?'

'Hmm,' I replied, frowning at him across the top of my wine glass. 'I don't want to do that – a load of doctors in white coats peering at me like I've gone mad.'

'I don't think it'll be like that,' he said, adopting that mock patient tone all blokes seem to be able to put on after a couple of decades of marriage.

'Well, I'll decide what I do about it,' I snapped.

'I'm sure you will,' he replied. 'As well as being the most

hardworking person I've ever met, you are of course also the most stubborn.'

He always said that. And, to be fair, he was right.

Over the next few days I went over and over what was going on with me. I didn't feel anxious all the time – it came and went in waves – but I knew that even when I was doing something I loved, like going for a walk or cooking, it could reappear at any moment. It was sort of there, beneath the surface, like the muddy depths beneath a still pond.

The only thing I could think of that might be causing the change in the way I was feeling was age and the menopause. I had had what were perhaps periods of depression in my forties and early fifties when the stress of working flat out on breakfast TV combined with caring for my mum and children all became a bit too much for me, but I'd never consulted a doctor about how I felt. In fact, I'd never go to the GP unless one of my limbs was falling off – I didn't like them and I was dead set against popping pills! So I muddled through those periods of depression and I was kind of OK. It was only when I hit fifty-five or fifty-six that I started to really feel not myself. I knew that was quite late for menopause – most women's periods stop when they're about fifty and that's when they notice other symptoms such as hot flushes, difficulty in sleeping, dry or itchy skin, weight gain and brain fog.

I'd been lucky and dodged some of the worst symptoms. The hot flushes could be annoying, but at least they were manageable and my weight was stable. All my adult life I'd been a size eight, despite my only exercise being the occasional brisk walk around the common. As for mood swings? Well, it's hard to spot them in yourself. There were times when I'd completely lose it with Martin and the boys, but tell me which woman doesn't lose her rag when living with three big men who still can't work out where to hang a wet towel or leave their trainers?

The worst menopause symptom was without doubt the brain fog. I'd be chatting away to Martin or a friend and then have no idea how the sentence was going to end. Or if I was out, I'd forget whether I'd brought my door key. I'd check my handbag and it would be there but ten minutes later, I'd have to check again. It was so frustrating. But so many women in their fifties complain of brain fog, I just had to hope it would pass.

I spent hours googling menopause symptoms and brain fog. Everything I read appeared to confirm what I was already thinking. There were stories from other women who seemed to be suffering exactly the same things as me – being unable to recall the name of someone I was talking about or walking into a room then forgetting why I was there or going to Tesco and returning home with half the things I needed. But because it was all happening so frequently now, it was making me anxious.

Deep down, I knew I had more reason than most to worry. My family history was littered with Alzheimer's disease. For years my greatest fear had been that one day it might come for me. But the more the brain fog persisted, the less I considered

Alzheimer's might be the cause. I was convinced it was the menopause.

Maybe I did need some heavy-duty hormone replacement therapy (HRT) or something that might ease the symptoms, untangle the knots in my brain and get me back on track?

Back to work . . .

2

I've never understood people who don't like to work. I've always loved it. I love feeling useful, achieving something each day, and let's be honest, I enjoyed earning the money too. It meant I could live my life the way I wanted to without being dependent on anyone. I guess my strong work ethic and craving for independence all come from my dad, Phil.

I want to tell you about Phil and my mum, Amy, so you can understand a bit more about me. We're all shaped by the major characters in our earliest years, maybe me more than most. I remained very close to my parents right up until they passed away – Mum in 2006 and Dad six years later. I wonder if that's maybe because on some deep level I understood my life would be shadowed by Alzheimer's too. Maybe I needed to be close to the problem.

Also, I think you need to understand who I was so you can see the impact this illness has had on me. And, to be honest, I find remembering my childhood way easier than the events of the past few years. I can tell stories of our mad dog Rufus escaping out to sea when we lived near Brighton with absolute clarity. I can even tell you the colour of his collar – blue. But here today I sometimes look out of the window and I can't even remember what season it is. Is it spring or autumn out there? And that's not just because it seems to always be raining!

Fifteen years ago, after Mum died, I wrote a book that told a lot of the story of my early life. This makes it easier now – it's like a crutch for my memory to lean upon. But there are still parts of my childhood, my working life and being a mum that remain crystal-clear. I want to share my memories with you, as best as I can, so you know what came to pass before I was struck by Alzheimer's. It's so important for me – and for all of us coping with this illness – to be more than just our diagnosis.

So yes, let me tell you what I remember about my life . . .

Dad's real name wasn't Phil – Phil Phillips would have been a bit mad, wouldn't it?! He was christened Neville when he was born in 1934, but when Tory Neville Chamberlain became prime minister three years later his raving socialist mum, Edith, refused to ever use the name again. So Phil it was.

He had a pretty tough childhood with a no-nonsense mother in a working-class area of Sheffield. I think the word 'battleaxe' was probably created for women of that generation, but I guess they needed to be strong to survive, bringing up kids while the men were away serving in the Second World War. After the war, the family moved all over the place; to Germany, Egypt, Malta and Scotland, following Grandad Reginald, who was a warrant officer in the British Army.

Maybe it was the constant moving in his childhood and being thrown into different schools that made Dad always feel like an outsider with few close friends and a deep disregard for authority. Grandma Edith always said he was a stubborn child or, to use her words, 'a little devil'. Hmm . . . I wonder if anyone else inherited that stubborn streak?

Grandad's dream was that Dad would follow him into the army so you can imagine how much of a 'devil' they thought he was when at eighteen he signed up for the navy instead. Dad joined the Royal Navy Fleet Air Arm and while the navy gave him the freedom to travel, it probably wasn't the best place for someone who had issues with authority. His application to become a pilot was rejected because of 'attitude'.

Later, he would tell us kids how, if only he'd had the chance, he could have been a pilot or a policeman or a teacher. There were to be a lot of 'if only's from my dad as he got older and more bitter about how his life had turned out.

What he did do after he left the navy in 1960 was fix TVs, which was a good job. I thought it was the best job in the world – who wants a TV that doesn't work? But Dad seemed increasingly frustrated that he hadn't achieved his dreams. He had no end of people to blame for his failures – Mum, us kids, 'them' in authority, society, you name it. In reality, the only person he had to blame was himself.

It was when he was based with the Fleet Air Arm at Haverfordwest in Pembrokeshire, West Wales, that he met twenty-six-year-old Eleanor Morris as she then was – before her entire identity became 'Mum'. Eleanor was known by her middle name, Amy, and she was out with friends at a dance at the local Masonic Hall when Dad and some of his mates turned up. She too had a fearsomely strict mother whose life's work was to protect the virtue of my mum and her four sisters.

Anyone who ever met Mum would talk about her wonderful, wide smile. After Dad died, I found some notes he'd made in his house. I had tears in my eyes when I read what he had written – but never told us – about meeting Mum: 'I saw her at a dance. Her and her dazzling smile. She's mine, I thought.'

Mum was the seventh of eight children from a tiny village called Dwrbach in Pembrokeshire. My grandma Mam Noddfa (Noddfa was the name of the house where she lived) had been twice-widowed by her mid-forties and was left alone to bring up all those children.

At fourteen, Mum had had to leave school and start work to help support the family. Later in life she'd laugh and say she'd always been 'tup', which was the Welsh way of saying stupid. That couldn't have been further from the truth. She might not have had a long list of qualifications, but she could talk to anyone and instinctively read situations and people; she had a warmth that meant everyone who met her loved her. And she was lovely to everyone. But she wasn't a pushover – she knew who she didn't like or who needed to be watched. And she was always right.

There had been sadness and trauma in Mum's childhood and later I wondered if that might have sparked the depression that blighted her final years. Her dad had died when she was very young and he was still only in his forties. And then, when she was fourteen, she was sexually assaulted by a local pig farmer while out playing in fields.

It was the 1940s and there was absolutely no thought that the crime would be reported to the police. The shame of such a thing was so great it wasn't even discussed. Even years later, when I was a teenager, Mum could never talk about it. Instead, I picked it up through half-stories and listening in on her chats with my aunties. Mostly, though, I think I learned about it from the sense of shame that seemed to emanate from Mum, particularly when it came to anything to do with sex.

She'd warn me if I wasn't 'tidy' (the Welsh way of saying respectable) then I'd get 'dragged'. For me growing up in Brighton, what did 'dragged' even mean? But I really didn't need to be told. The sense of menace of that word coupled with the message that if this were to happen it would be all my fault said it all.

Later, when I was old enough to think it through, it broke my heart. All her life my mum was so kind, so chatty and giggly, so sweet and with an incredible innocence, but beneath all that she clearly still carried a sense of being dirty and shameful.

Mum had worked in a draper's store in Fishguard before training as a nurse. She was working as a nurse that evening she went to the dance and met Dad. And the rest, as they say, is history.

My history.

Within months, Dad had left the navy and moved to Canterbury in Kent, where Mum soon joined him for their wedding on 26 March 1960 at St Paul's Church in the city. I don't think their relationship was ever plain sailing. Dad even went missing for a couple of days after they first got engaged – goodness only knows why he did it or where he went. But despite all that, somehow their relationship worked. As a married couple, they lodged in a two-bed Victorian terraced house with a widow called Mrs Wilson. Then, just a smidge over nine months after their wedding, I arrived on New Year's Day 1961.

Dad really wasn't ready for me. How do I know? Well, somehow over the years Mum told me the whole story: how he'd been so shocked when he found out she was pregnant that he made her go to the doctor and ask about an abortion. I don't really know how Mum felt about that, but I do know the local doctor sent her home with some Valium and a few stern words for Dad.

He must have come around in the end, I guess, or maybe he just accepted it as his lot? It's a strange story to know about your entry into the world, though, isn't it? Would it have been better if I'd never known? Probably. But in later years, when Mum was depressed and upset, those little insights into her life and marriage that were kept so tightly shrouded in secrecy for years gradually began to emerge. Like how he'd never turned up at my christening. Mum's entire family and Dad's parents were all in the photos, gathered around me in my white satin gown, but Dad was nowhere to be seen – he'd just upped and gone again.

Still, he reappeared at some point – I'm not sure when or where he went – and they must have muddled through because twenty months after I was born, my brother David turned up. By then we'd moved into new digs in a nearby council house with Mrs Wilson, or 'Narnie' as us kids knew her. Dad always said, 'She thinks she's the Queen of Sheba,' but Narnie was like a parent to Mum and Dad, and a loving but strict granny to me and David.

My earliest memories are of that house, of Narnie and her blue-rinse hair (what was that colour all about?), her peep-toe heels and a confected accent that made her appear a bit posher than the late Queen Elizabeth. I think it was Narnie who taught Mum how to look after two demanding little kids and a frequently difficult husband – but like so many women of that era, Narnie could also be fiercely critical and judgemental of other women.

Poor Mum must have felt she was constantly under attack for some perceived failing in her life, be it from Narnie, her own mum, her mother-in-law or her husband. And while I was way too young to realize it at the time, maybe this had an impact on her mental health.

The phrase 'mental health' hadn't even been invented in the 1960s. Mum would just call it 'trouble with my nerves', but my brother and I could tell when she was struggling. She went from being so warm and loving to becoming withdrawn and snapping at me and David for no reason. And every couple of months she would suffer crippling migraines that made her physically sick. Us kids would be left to play in the front room while she shut herself away in her bedroom with the curtains closed. It felt like it went on for days on end.

The joke in our family was that Dad worked in TV long before I did. There was nothing he couldn't tell you about transistors, resistors and circuit boards. And while fixing televisions is very much a land-locked job, he never lost his need to be free, which he must have found in the navy. He was constantly away fixing televisions, sometimes for days on end. Christmas was particularly busy when everyone wanted their tellies working in time for *The Morecambe and Wise Show* or *Val Doonican*. Most were still black and white – only the well-off had a colour TV – and they were so expensive that everyone hired them from the rental shop Rediffusion, where Dad worked. All day he'd dash around from one job to the next, then come home completely exhausted, sit on the sofa and watch telly.

I don't think my brother David and I were left in much doubt that Dad preferred television to us. It was a different time though and dads back then didn't spend hours playing with their kids or taking them to clubs and playdates like they do nowadays. They are much more hands-on these days. Back then, dads went to work and brought in the money while mums stayed at home. Our dad was particularly driven by the need to earn enough for us to move out of Narnie's and into our own house.

When David was about three and I was five, Dad did it. He'd got enough for us to buy a three-bed semi with a pillar-box red front door in St Stephen's Close, Canterbury. Soon after, we had our very own car too – a bright red Mini parked out the front. We'd become like one of those 'proper' families we saw on one of Dad's TVs.

Dad was incredibly proud of what he'd achieved through sheer, hard graft. Neither of my parents had the luxury of the

Bank of Mum and Dad – they did everything themselves – and for an independent man like my father that meant everything.

But getting on the housing ladder just made Dad work even harder for all the 'mod cons' a family of that time needed – a three-piece suite, a fitted carpet, and if we were really going up in the world, an avocado-coloured fitted bathroom! And so he only really passed fleetingly through our lives, getting in from work as we went up to bed or sitting in the chair on a Sunday afternoon. Everything else was work, which meant all the burden of organizing our family life fell on Mum. It must have been lonely and exhausting for her with Dad rarely there and us kids constantly messing around, fighting and generally causing carnage.

But for us it was a pretty idyllic life. When David was still in the pushchair, I'd walk alongside as Mum pushed, stopping to chat to absolutely everyone she met. She'd say it was a Welsh thing, but everyone loved her because she was so chatty. 'What a lovely day,' she'd comment to a total stranger as we passed them in the street. Half an hour later, she would still be talking to them, having extracted their life story and commiserated or congratulated them on everything they had going on. It drove me and David mad although as I grew older and was dragged around on Mum's trips for cups of tea with her friends in the afternoon after they'd finished the housework, I started to enjoy listening to the women's conversations; the laughter, the stories shared and the gossip exchanged. For me it was like a tiny window into what women really thought.

David and I had loads of friends who lived in our close and

we'd play with them after school and during those long summer holidays. Being so near in age meant we always had someone to hang around with – when we weren't fighting! On hot days we would walk down to the bottom of the close, across the main road and down to the River Stour, laden with yellow fishing nets, buckets, Mum's old jam jars and the absolute certainty we were about to catch our dinner. Much to Mum's disgust, we'd return home with eels and all sorts of tiny fish, then have to take them all back to the river the next morning.

There may not be many five-year-olds nowadays who can read a knitting pattern for baby booties or the recipe for a hearty mid-week chicken casserole, but I could! Because I pretty much learned to read from studying the pages of Mum's *Woman* and *Woman's Own* magazines. We weren't one of those homes with shelves lined with books – although Dad was very proud of his *Encyclopedia Britannica* – but from an early age I loved absorbing new information. And if that was the problem page of *Woman's Own*, then so be it!

Dad had bought me the *Peter and Jane* Ladybird books with their lovely pictures of a brother and sister just like me and David (without the wrestling and screaming and wailing!) when I was first trying to put together sentences. Like so many men a bit frustrated with their daily life, Dad loved books and the idea that they could transport you to another world, but perhaps also like others who feel their life hasn't matched their dreams, he put pressure on me to do better. When my friends' dads bought them copies of *Bunty* magazine, my dad came home with copies of *Look and Learn*: 'If you read, you can learn anything,' he'd say. And he was right. He was adamant that education was the jet plane to a better, independent life and he was determined that my brother and I should be educated and, of course, be independent.

At first, that went well. I was still at junior school when I won a national poetry competition run by Brooke Bond Tea and I'd be the girl made to stand up in assembly to read out my latest story or poem. By the age of six I had a reading age of eleven. I still messed around and had a 'silly streak' as my school report said, but I loved reading and so learning came easily to me. And it turned out that Dad was absolutely right – my love of reading and discovering information became my passport to a career in journalism.

3

I was seven and David was five when Dad was promoted by Rediffusion to a new job in Brighton and we all moved down to the Sussex coast.

By then David and I were inseparable. All these years on, our lives have taken us in different directions with different family responsibilities, but we remain close and speak frequently on the phone. I love it when he comes to visit and he is someone with whom I can share those memories of childhood – who is able to help keep them alive for me. It seems important to share memories of a long time ago – of the time before Alzheimer's – and it is comforting that my brother knows the real me, the person I was.

When we arrived on the South Coast, it was 1968. The two piers stretched out into the sea and the Brighton seafront was a dazzling mix of arcades, bars with crazily dressed people pouring out, cockle sheds and loud music. The Mods and Rockers gangs with their scooters and leather jackets might have gone but there was still an edgy, brash feel to the place. Even I could sense that at seven. It couldn't have been any more exciting.

Except we didn't actually live in Brighton. We were a couple of miles down the coast in a little town called Peacehaven, where the only scooters were mobility scooters and the only dancing was at the OAPs' tea dance. It lacked the grit and glamour of Brighton, but had neatly trimmed gardens and net curtains in abundance.

I was sent to Telscombe Cliffs Junior School, which was a struggle at first. All the other girls already had 'best friends for ever' and scented rubbers with those words stamped on them to prove it. I spent at least a year faking all sorts of stomach bugs and sickness to get out of going there. I thought I'd fooled Mum good and proper about what was really going on, but maybe she knew and was waiting for me to fit in in my own good time.

In many ways David remained my best friend. We were entirely left to our own devices while Mum cooked, cleaned and chatted on her daily trips to the shops. Now instead of the river, David and I had the South Downs to roam in our spare time. It wouldn't happen now, but we were allowed out by ourselves to explore every inch of the Downs. Looking back, I sometimes think our life was a bit like one of Enid Blyton's *Famous Five* books. We even had our very own four-legged best friend – Rufus – whom Mum and Dad bought soon after we moved to Brighton. He was a 'thoroughbred Beagle', Mum would tell anyone who stopped to chat above the noise of his endless yapping. The rest of his time was spent trying to dig his way out of the garden.

Rufus's life was like a feature-length screening of *The Great*

Escape. We once found him high up on the cliffs overlooking the English Channel. Another time the Fire Brigade had to rescue him from the sea because he'd found his way down to the beach and become stranded. The worst, though, was the day when Mum and I got stuck in a traffic jam on the A23 and were grumbling about what was causing the big hold-up . . . only for us to get to the front of the queue to see Rufus in the middle of the road, furiously barking at cars!

Even in our new home, Dad was just as busy and absent from our lives as he had ever been. Years later, when I had a husband and children of my own, I wondered why Mum never put her foot down about his ability to disappear from family life for most of the week, but she seemed to completely hero-worship him: 'You should be grateful for how hard your dad works to look after us,' she would say. Or, 'He's such a clever man, your dad – there's nothing he can't fix.' Why it didn't drive her berserk that he never got around to fixing anything in our house and just slumped in front of the telly exhausted all the time when he did come home, I really don't know.

When I was still at junior school, about nine years old, Dad worked himself so hard that he became rundown and ended up in hospital with viral pneumonia. It took Mum an hour on the bus to get to the isolation hospital and she was desperately worried about him. I don't think David and I really understood at first what was going on – or certainly not how serious it was going to be.

One evening, after we had gone to bed, I heard Mum crying on the phone downstairs. 'How long will it take you to get here?' she was saying. 'You need to be quick.' And at that moment I realized just how bad it was. Mum was pleading for Dad's parents – who were then running a pub in Canterbury – to come quickly as the hospital was saying he had become gravely ill.

Seeing Mum crying in the hall was frightening.

In the end, Dad pulled through.

'The stubborn bugger,' said Grandma, who'd updated the 'little devil' nickname for her son.

Not that she was wrong. He *was* a stubborn bugger.

Which probably didn't help Mum in those years. As David and I got older, her headaches kept returning. While much of the time she was still the same chatty woman she had always been, other days it was as if a darkness descended on her. She would seem so sad and fragile, like everything had become too much. Since I was tiny she'd always called me 'Toots'. Mum was so loving and warm to be around, but when she had her dark days there wasn't anything even her 'little Toots' could do to lift her. And there's no doubt, with Dad rarely anywhere to be seen, David and I could become too much.

We loved to fight. One of us would wind up the other and off we'd go. By then I was becoming as stubborn as my dad and would never give in to my younger brother – and David just loved causing trouble.

One afternoon we had been wrestling around the front room when David whacked me with the iron poker from the coal fire. I screamed as the pain juddered through my head. Mum just totally lost it. She rang Dad at work to say she'd had enough, but she got no sympathy from him: 'What are you ringing me for?' he said.

I think something snapped in Mum that day. She put on her coat and stormed off to the bus stop. David and I couldn't believe it and ran after her, begging her to come back. Surely our mum, the kindest, loveliest person in the world, wouldn't leave us? But she jumped on the bus to Brighton and that was it – we were left with our own sickening sense of guilt. Not to mention my throbbing head.

Of course she did come back, but something had changed. I think Mum realized she deserved more from life than just being a slave to her husband and kids. She got a job behind the bar at a nearby Butlin's in Saltdean. But Dad didn't like the idea of his wife working behind a bar and, whether it was that or the difficulty juggling work with having to do everything else for the family, she packed the job in after a short while.

And whether Mum liked it or not, the Phillips family was soon on the move again – this time to Southampton after Dad got promoted 'to management', as Mum would boast, for a new TV rental company called Telefusion. Again, David and I went through the childhood trauma of joining new schools, where we definitely felt like the odd kids out. Not helped by Mum deciding she'd knit me a skirt in bottle green for my school uniform. I mean a knitted skirt? I might as well have had a sign above my head saying 'bully me'. And they did. There were some tough kids at Aldermoor Middle School and the half-mile walk there and back was like taking your life in your hands. Several times I was picked on by older boys walking home. They'd push me over and kick me when I was on the floor. It sounds barbaric now, but that's how things were then if your face didn't fit. I'd return home with cuts and grazes on my hands and knees, and dust all over my knitted skirt. I don't know whether Mum didn't notice or simply turned a blind eye, or I just managed to hide my injuries from her. I couldn't have told her – it would have upset her too much. It's funny, isn't it, that even as a child you know just how much you can let a parent worry about you?

Gradually, though, I settled in and made a few friends, but I'd changed a lot from the little girl who was winning prizes for her poetry. I didn't want to be an outsider, I wanted to fit in – and if that meant messing around with some of the other girls, that's exactly what I did.

I was in and out of the headteacher's office for the cane across my hand for general messing around. It stung like crazy, but I bit my lip. My dad's stubborn streak was now in full effect and I wasn't going to let anyone, particularly the headteacher, think they'd got the better of me.

Mum was going potty, thinking I was 'going off the rails', and – I don't know whether she insisted or the teachers thought it was for the best – I was moved into a different class, where it was decided I wouldn't be so 'easily led'. It was there that I became best friends with Debbie. She lived in our road, but we hadn't really talked much as I'd been putting all my efforts into fitting in with the cool kids.

Soon, though, Debs and I were together all the time.

It was around about then that I got my first big job in the media. Yep, I was a papergirl for the *Southampton Evening Echo*! Everyone got the *Echo* back then and I'd whizz around the streets on my bike, shoving copies through letterboxes as if I was in a race against time. I was only eleven, but I loved the idea I had a job – and loved earning my own money even more. It was seventy-five pence a week for going out every evening and then a bit more for the Sunday morning round. OK, not a fortune but like my dad had always told me, it meant I was independent. And if I wanted a dress or some flares from Mum's Great Universal catalogue, I could buy them, especially when they were only ever something like fifty pence a week for a million weeks!

After a while, I started doing a Littlewoods Pools round too. I seemed to have more than my fair share of dirty old men on my round, but I learned to make sure I kept plenty of distance between myself and them – and I never stepped over the front step. I was determined I wasn't going to be getting 'dragged'.

With my paper round and now the Pools round too I felt like I'd won the Pools myself! I could go out shopping with Debs whenever I wanted or get my hair cut without having to ask for Mum and Dad's money – or permission.

Soon after, I got a job behind the counter in the paper shop. No one worried about whether I was old enough to be working at weekends and after school and it certainly didn't bother me. I felt quite the grown-up, handing over packets of chewing gum and cigarettes and then ringing up people's change on the electronic till. Except maybe I wasn't quite so mature as I'd thought I was. As I was about to find out . . .

Mum and her friend Auntie Joan (not a real auntie but all your mum's friends were aunties back then) had met up to go shopping and I was trailing along behind one Saturday afternoon. After a while we all trooped into Mothercare, where we never normally went. Mum and Joan started giggling over baby clothes, cots and high chairs and then, as if I'd been hit by a speeding train, I realized what was going on: Mum was pregnant. She'd been acting a bit strange for a while, there were whispered conversations between her and Dad and she'd put on a bit of weight around her tummy, but it hadn't occurred to me it could be that. Not that. Not a baby, at forty. Not my mum and dad having S-E-X. The whole thing felt utterly gross. Not only was I furious, I was also hurt that Mum had decided not to share this momentous secret with me but was quite happy to gossip and giggle about it with Auntie Joan.

As you may have picked up, we weren't a family that talked about feelings, and we certainly didn't talk about things such as where babies come from. Obviously, I'd worked that information out back at Telscombe Cliffs Junior School, but now, on the verge of becoming a teenager myself, I didn't want to be discussing it with my mum.

It was weeks later when Mum finally admitted to me and David that we had a new brother or sister on the way. David was equally appalled, but he got over things quicker. I was so mortified, I couldn't even face being seen with Mum.

One day she stood outside school waiting to fetch us, her

baby bump on full show, and I could feel a burning sense of shame.

'Toots,' she called out to me, but I pretended I couldn't hear and walked straight past her. She must have realized that I had seen her and was probably terribly hurt by me. But I was hurt too. Thankfully, when our little brother Andrew arrived on 28 December 1972, all our concerns evaporated. He was just gorgeous and we all adored him.

Mum had her hands full looking after the new baby and I worked more and more mornings and evenings at the news-agent's. I loved doing my best there, being super organised, tidying the newspapers and restocking the shelves the moment items were sold. Yes, I liked the money I was earning, but what I really loved was the actual work. I had such a great laugh with the other staff and they became like an extended family to me.

Work in the shop was also a sanctuary of calm compared to school.

Perhaps I should explain a bit more about that wild streak I'd once had. Sometimes I like to blame it on the 'bad influence' of the mates I made in the seniors at Millbrook School, but the truth is more likely the only person to blame was me.

Millbrook was rough. Properly rough. There were girls getting pregnant, boys being sent to Borstal, windows were smashed and really not much work was being done at all. From my early teens I had dreamed of being a doctor. I'm not sure if this was fuelled by a heartfelt passion to save lives or just those endless repeats of *Dr. Kildare* on TV. The big problem with the

whole doctor dream, though, was it meant getting high grades
– *very high* grades. Any chance of that was going rapidly out of
the window as I did my best to fit in at Millbrook – and fitting
in meant doing the least possible work to avoid being labelled
a 'swot' or a 'square'.

I was only thirteen when I started drinking regularly – and
heavily too. Dad was always at work and Mum was up to her
eyes looking after Andrew and keeping the house tidy so it was
actually quite easy to slip away in the evenings without being
noticed. My friends and I would buy barley wine from the
newsagent (it was the cheapest stuff available), smash the top
off on the kerb then take it to the youth club, where we'd
surreptitiously neck it in the corner. Or as some of the other
kids' parents really didn't care what they got up to, we'd go
around their houses and smoke and drink in their bedrooms
until we were sick.

Around then, I also became a massive Southampton fan and
would go to all the home games – and away matches too if I
could work it around my shifts at the newsagent. I once told
Mum and Dad I was going around my mate's for a sleepover
but was actually on the coach to Belgium to watch Southampton
against RSC Anderlecht in the European Cup Winners' Cup.
Still only sixteen, I got away with it! But I could afford it so
why shouldn't I? At least that's what my teenage brain was
telling me.

I guess getting through Millbrook without a long-lasting
drinking problem or a pregnancy was a result. Certainly, I had
no O-level results worth talking about. But even if I'd been a

bit silly for a few years, I wasn't stupid. I realized that if I had any hope of becoming a doctor, I needed to get some qualifications.

Debs and I moved to sixth form at Hill College for Girls, where I retook my failed O levels and an English A level, then added a couple more A levels in the second year. It was a calmer place with no boys to distract us from studying as Debs and I both tried to make up for lost time on our O levels.

Although just seventeen, I'd managed to get myself a very mature twenty-eight-year-old boyfriend. Mum and Dad were pretty relaxed about what I got up to by then and they knew they'd created an independent, stubborn young woman so really what chance did they have of trying to control me?

And then the real thing happened – first love. We met at the Top Rank club in Southampton. Joe was a goalie for Southampton, six foot tall, broad, muscly and just all-round gorgeous! For four and a half years he was the love of my life. He'd collect me from college in his Mk3 Ford Cortina and we'd go around mine for tea – Mum loved him too. Or sometimes we'd go out for a drink. Everything seemed so easy when he was around. Joe also provided security, which was important for me because around about then, Mum and Dad simply upped sticks and moved back to Wales with little Andrew. David and I were left pretty much on our own.

Maybe this was why Dad had wanted us to be independent.

4

Dad had fallen out with pretty much everyone at work and decided he wanted a new start. And if Dad decided something, the rest of us fitted in with his plans. At first he stayed on his own in a caravan in Tenby while he got a job (fixing televisions again) and a house. Then a few months later, Mum and Andrew joined him. Our family home in Southampton went on the market and Mum found me a room in the house of a lovely widow she knew while David moved in with one of our old teachers.

It sounds a bit shocking now that they upped and left their two teenage children alone in Southampton while they went to Wales, but at the time we just got on with it. Hopefully that's as good an example as any about how independent I was brought up to be. Parents of teenagers almost certainly couldn't imagine doing anything like that nowadays, but back then I just took it in my stride. I loved Mum and Dad, but I also knew I was more than capable of coping on my own. That's why the loss of independence and confidence I've suffered in recent years has been so difficult to come to terms with – it really isn't the natural 'me'.

I don't think Mum ever wanted to disappear back to Wales but, in reality, she probably didn't have much choice. It was never discussed, but I think we all knew that on some level Mum just had to do whatever Dad wanted.

I'm still not entirely certain what made the relationship between Mum and Dad tick. Or if it really did tick at all. More than once I heard Dad snap at Mum: 'I never loved you.' Then he made it into a family joke – was that to cover his shame at being so cruel to her or did he just think his marriage was a joke? I really don't know. Clearly, he was deeply frustrated at how life had turned out for him. He certainly spent a lot of his life dreaming. One of his big dreams was that as a family we would all move to South Africa and start a new life. But like so many dreamers, it was never his fault when the dreams went wrong. His version of why we never made it to South Africa was, 'That bloody woman wouldn't go without the dining-room table.'

'That bloody woman' was my lovely mum. And admittedly she did love that dining-room table she'd saved up for when they first married, but she'd have followed Dad to the ends of the earth (with or without a table). No, it was just another one of his excuses.

When I was still at junior school, there would be times I'd be tucked up in bed at night and would hear Mum and Dad rowing downstairs. Dad had a temper that could go from nought to a hundred in a matter of moments. Once we were all sitting around that infamous dining table and he totally lost it and rapped Mum's hands with a spoon. That must have really hurt, but we all just pretended it hadn't happened – horrible, really.

'Don't ever get married, Fiona,' Dad would tell me.

I thought I never would – it certainly didn't seem to be a barrel of laughs. I don't really understand what he truly felt about us kids either, but I do know he focused every fibre of his being into giving us all the best life he could. He hated the idea of being dependent on anyone for anything or being in debt to someone, and he worked so hard to prevent that. For him, independence was the greatest achievement. And I guess I, his devoted follower, just absorbed that from him: to be independent was the mission. Which is why I was determined to do something that mattered with my life – but something that would also give me financial and emotional independence.

Although I had done quite well in my A levels, I realized my dream of becoming a doctor was just that – a dream. Instead I thought I'd try training as a radiographer. It felt like the closest thing I could find to being a doctor without the seven years at medical school. But that didn't last long. I hadn't realized the job really just meant pressing a few buttons and then looking at X-rays – there were none of the fun bits like talking to patients and assessing their needs.

After a year in the role I jacked it in. By then it was 1980, Mrs Thatcher and her Conservative government were in power and the country was lurching towards one of the worst periods of unemployment in its history. Jobs were few and far between. The best I could find was in a Mr Kipling factory, where my responsibility was sorting between the perfect and not-so-perfect cakes. That lasted just weeks before I packed it in again and decided to apply for university.

It was around this time that Alzheimer's first touched my life. Before then, I was probably like a lot of people in those days whose only understanding of dementia was that old people went a bit ga-ga at some point. There was never any thought about why that might be or what could be done to prevent it or make their lives better and more dignified.

I was a student filled with that youthful sense of certainty that such a thing would never happen to me. I was too invincible to be old. Or sick. At least I think it was Alzheimer's that struck down Dad's mum, my grandma, but we never really talked properly about what was going on. It's not that long ago – only the early 1980s – but Alzheimer's disease still wasn't being properly discussed. It felt like there was some secret shame surrounding it.

For years before they retired, Grandma and Grandad had run a pub in Canterbury. Grandma – who as I've said was a proper battleaxe – had always been obsessive about cleanliness and there can never have been a more spick-and-span pub, but after they retired, she became forgetful and withdrawn. And she couldn't keep on top of the cleaning in their little flat. For ages I thought it was simply old age. Then I went over to visit and noticed Grandma had laid out framed photos of her three children – Dad, Uncle Barry and Auntie Germaine – and put piles of sweets next to the three of them.

'What are the sweets doing, Grandma?' I asked.

'Oh, that's just in case they get hungry,' she said.

'Well, that's very kind,' I laughed.

At first I thought she must be getting a touch of confusion – I still didn't think my tough-as-old-boots grandma had anything more serious than that. I didn't realize she was losing her grip on the world or that it wouldn't be returning. And of course Mum and Dad didn't discuss it. 'Oh, your grandma just gets a bit muddled sometimes' was as far as the conversation went. It was another of those things that went unremarked in our family. Undiscussed.

Untouched.

Then Grandma was diagnosed with cervical cancer but, by the time she passed away, a couple of years later, her mind was totally gone.

What a tragedy. Alzheimer's would return to take the memories and lives of two of Grandma's three children – Dad and my Uncle Barry. And then, of course, it has returned for me. If I'd known back then, aged nineteen, that one day I would end up with the same illness as my grandma, would I have done things differently? I don't think so. And although now there is much talk of tests that will tell people years in advance whether it's likely they'll be hit by the disease, I would never have wanted to know.

Back then, I was confident and excited and I felt nothing could get in the way of living the independent adult life ahead of me – I'm glad I didn't know how it would play out. It was that desire to get out and see the world that made me accept an offer to study English at Birmingham Uni. Joe had moved to the Midlands to play for a First Division side, which was a huge achievement, and going to Birmingham meant I would be able to see him at weekends.

Every weekend we were like an old married couple – shopping, cooking and watching TV. It started to feel a bit too grown-up and I wonder if it also meant I never really threw myself into student life either. I felt as though everyone else was a lot younger than me – I suppose they were. But it added to the sense that I was becoming trapped in a steady relationship just as my uni friends were waiting for life to begin.

I still loved Joe, but once more the need to be independent and free overwhelmed everything. By the time I'd graduated, at twenty-three, my first love might have been over, but it felt as though there were still many adventures ahead. I'd got the idea – I'm really not sure where from – that I would like to be a journalist. I loved English and reading and I was curious about the world, all skills that make for a good journalist. But I was worried. It was a lot of money to study for a postgraduate broadcasting course in London. Despite a string of casual jobs, I didn't have enough and I couldn't ask Mum and Dad to fund it.

My brother David and I spent a summer living in the South of France, staying in a grungy campsite and selling doughnuts on nudist beaches. Yes, that was me; that was the sort of thing I did when I was young. I wasn't careless, but I was carefree – I wasn't anxious about things, life was just a huge adventure that was there for the taking. The difference in the way I feel today is almost overwhelming.

Those crazy days were huge fun and I did earn a little money – enough to keep us in baguettes and red wine – but it was nowhere near what I needed for the broadcasting course. Then someone suggested I apply for a grant from the Catherine and Lady Grace James Foundation, which helped young Welsh people struggling to meet the costs of postgraduate studies. That was a life-changing moment – without the philanthropy of the James family my life might have been very different.

I applied to – and was accepted at – the National Broadcasting School in Soho, London, where I learned the skills of being a reporter. But really there's only one skill that job needs – the ability to talk and listen to anyone and everyone. A skill I'd been learning from Mum since the day I was born.

The big-time job I'd hoped for on the BBC or ITV after graduating wasn't easy to come by though. I applied for dozens and dozens of jobs with no luck. After a couple more spells grape picking in France and working in a Soho fish and chip shop, I finally got a break.

Admittedly this was not the big time but I was in the door! My job was writing and reading the runners and riders guide for the William Hill Racing phone line. From there, I went on to AA Roadwatch, which provided the traffic reports for radio stations across London and the South East.

I hoped that appearing on so many radio stations would one day lead to a reporter job on one of them. All the while I never stopped working, trying to improve, trying to show how much I wanted the next step. The work ethic I'd inherited from Dad was as strong as ever – I just wanted the chance to prove myself at the next stage.

Sure enough, the chance came when I was offered weekend reporting shifts at County Sound radio in Guildford, Surrey, and the work just kept coming in. And that damned work ethic meant I could never say 'no' to an opportunity either!

For about eight years I took every bit of work I could lay my hands on. Sometimes I was getting up at 2 a.m., driving to Peterborough for the breakfast show and returning for the drive-time programme in Surrey. Then doing it all over again the next day.

It was through AA Roadwatch that I heard there was a hunt on for a presenter for a regional TV show in Norfolk called *Weekend*. I was terrified going for the screen test. Everyone else in the waiting room seemed so much more experienced, beautiful and polished than me. I couldn't believe it when back home in my London flat, I got the call to say I'd got the job – it was so exciting.

TV, here I come!

At that point I only became more frantic about work – I could see exactly how competitive I had to be in order to succeed. As well as the Norfolk presenting role, I took on reporting shifts at Sky News. Anything to build up my experience and get myself noticed in this cut-throat world. Finally, all the hard work led me to some reporting shifts on *GMTV*, the new morning breakfast show, in 1993.

It had been a bumpy start for the show, which took over from the much-loved TV-am show *Good Morning Britain* – it was essential we made it work and earned the trust of the British breakfast-eating public.

5

So that's the bit of my life up until landing my first job at *GMTV*. It feels a million miles away now, yet some of those memories are still so vivid. Like the evenings Debs and I would go dancing at the Top Rank. Or the days when my brother David and I went fishing in that river with our nets on bamboo rods.

Other bits of my story have been harder to retell and I've had to rely on memories I've written about before or interviews I've done over the years about my childhood. I've also talked to my family and friends about those days. I'm aware that there are plenty of parts of my childhood that I can't properly recall now, but then who can remember much about their childhood beyond a few standout moments, seconds in time that have stuck in the mind? And more often than not those moments are the ones that were captured on your mum's Kodak Instamatic camera or have become a favourite family story, retold dozens of times, rather than things you truly remember. Can any of us really recall one specific moment from fifty years ago unless it was something completely shocking or traumatic?

How reliable is any memory anyway? We smile as we look at the snap of the family huddled around a flask of tea, grinning for the camera, and think we recall what a lovely day we had back then. But we forget the niggling that had gone on all morning as everyone rushed around, trying to find the flask in the top cupboard, arguing about whether to take the A27 or the B-roads with a better view but more potholes. Or how we moaned about the drizzle making our hair go frizzy or how Dad got angry because someone spilt a can of Pepsi on his back-seat upholstery. So many memories are filtered and fudged by pictures or the perceptions of others.

Experts say most people remember nothing before the age of three. And only momentous events – or a general sense of a person or place, rather than a precise moment – before we reach ten. Our memories are selective as to what we keep – and what we discard. Scientists reckon if it wasn't that way women would never have more than one baby! If we truly remembered the pain of our first child, who would go back for a second? But instead we recall the warm, wonderful moments when we first hold a baby – and that wipes out all the bad bits.

I guess my mind is just being more selective than most now.

The memories I hold onto are when Mum, Dad, me, David and then later, Andrew, were together and things were good. I know all too well it wasn't always great in our family, but it's the good that lasts. It's a sense of being loved that remains long after precise memories have gone.

I can't remember a specific moment when Mum sat me on

her lap and read me a story when I was tiny or kissed me good-night. Or hugged me when I went off to university. And I can't remember every time Dad gave me a satisfied nod and a pat on the back when I came home from the newsagent with my neatly folded (small) pile of pound notes I'd earned that week. But they definitely happened because my memory knows – *I* know – how much I was loved by Mum and how much I made my dad proud. It's those memories – most of which are lost to me now – that must still live on somewhere inside me because they shaped the person I became and guided every decision I have made.

When we are little there's just a handful of people making those memories that bury into us for life; maybe a mum, dad and a couple of teachers. But as we get older, there are so many more people – best mates like my friend Debs, boyfriends like Joe and then the people you meet through work. And all of those times, good and bad, with those people are the building blocks of who you become. I try to comfort myself by thinking that, even though I might not remember lots of those times now, they must still be inside me somewhere – because they made me.

By the end of this book, you will still have these stories, but I may not. You'll know more about me than I do! That's a joke by the way – thank God I can still laugh about this awful situation. But knowing I'm losing these memories hurts too. Of course it bloody does! But that's where I'm at. As Dad would say, 'No point in moaning, just got to get on with it.'

So back to it. And with help from old newspaper cuttings and TV clips that you can still find on YouTube, let me tell you what happened when I first made my way into the bright, shiny world of television.

6

Finally, I was on a TV show that transmitted beyond Norfolk – and even as far as Wales. My role on *GMTV* was as a general reporter, which meant if there was a snowstorm or a bus crash, a court case or a haul of Roman coins discovered, then I was the one who'd be dispatched to the scene. And I loved it. The call would usually come in the evening and then I'd be off straight away to wherever I was needed to start reporting at the crack of dawn. It was tough, but for me it never felt like hard work because I loved talking to people. It was fun. I laughed a lot and it seemed I had the 'bubbly' kind of personality that TV liked.

'Bubbly' sounds like one of those terribly nineties clichés, but what television needs is people with enthusiasm and energy. And because I was so incredibly grateful to be there, I had those in bucketloads.

Mum and Dad were bursting with pride. There can't have been anyone in the whole of Pembrokeshire who didn't know what Amy Phillips' daughter was up to at that point. We were once in the queue at Tesco in Haverfordwest when Mum tapped the woman in front of us on the shoulder and said: 'This is my daughter, Fiona. She's on *GMTV*, you know.' I was mortified and wanted to climb inside the checkout conveyor belt, but that didn't bother Mum. She'd always been unbelievably chatty with everyone she met, but to me it felt like her willingness to strike up a conversation anywhere was becoming almost a bit eccentric.

Although Mum couldn't help but boast about me and her 'brilliant actor' son David (who was working in theatre in London), she was keen to listen to other peoples' stories too. She was always curious – some might say nosey – about the people she met. In another time and place she would have made an incredible journalist.

My determination to make any assignment that I was sent on work well soon led to an amazing opportunity – the chance to cover the 1993 Oscars ceremony. I couldn't believe my luck. I'd actually be in Hollywood on the red carpet (well, reporting along the red carpet anyway). It was more than I could have ever dreamed of just a few years earlier.

Maybe I should have felt apprehensive when I stood at Heathrow airport waiting to board that flight to Los Angeles. But I didn't – I couldn't wait to get there.

When I'm with friends now, one of the things I talk about most is memories of those first few weeks in LA. It was such a huge adventure for a girl from a very normal family in a very normal street, who went to a very normal school, to suddenly find herself in the global centre of glamour. It was such a shock to the system and maybe that's why the memories of this time remain with me more vividly than other experiences. It was a truly happy time too. If you picture me – the brave, adventurous, having-a-ball me, rather than the me I've become through illness – maybe think of me driving my soft-top car down Sunset Boulevard.

When I arrived in LA that first time, I dropped my bags at my hotel and then set off for the Beverly Hills Hotel, where I was due to meet Neal Harrison, who was to be my producer on the job – so the guy who would help me set up interviews and get the work done.

As soon as I sat down at the table opposite Neal, we clicked. We made each other laugh, but we clearly both loved work and were driven to do the best possible job that we could. We both had loads of ideas about the celebrities we wanted to get on camera as they emerged from the Oscars ceremony. It was a great meeting, but I don't think either of us that day had any idea that we were starting a friendship that would last for the rest of our lives. Neal is one of the people helping me write this book now, helping me recover the memories of that period and hold those great times we shared in my mind once again.

The actual Oscars ceremony didn't go as well as we had hoped. There was a problem with the cable to our cameras, which meant we were further than we wanted to be from the red carpet that the celebrities walked up and down. So, instead of just casually calling them over for a chat, I had to keep running backwards and forwards to persuade them to walk four minutes out of their way to where our camera was positioned.

Nothing on earth was going to prevent me from snaffling some good celebrities though. This was my big moment. I'd been entrusted with the job because the bosses knew I could talk to anyone – I couldn't let them or the viewers watching live in London down. I managed to persuade Gene Hackman, who'd won Best Supporting Actor, and Clint Eastwood, who'd won Best Director for the Western *Unforgiven*, to come over to talk to us.

Afterwards, the editors in London were thrilled that we had managed to land two actual Oscar winners, but Neal and I were just disappointed we hadn't been able to catch even more celebrities. We both vowed that if we got the chance to report on the Academy Awards again we would make sure *everyone* stopped to talk to us.

Our editor in London wanted me to stay out in Los Angeles to do a fun feature with the model who had been Julia Roberts' legs double in the movie *Pretty Woman*. It was hilarious. We all – me, Neal and the model – went up and down Rodeo Drive, strolling through the Gucci boutique and all the other designer stores and getting stared at by shoppers as if we were completely mad. How could it be possible that this was a job and I was getting paid for having so much fun?

I returned home to London, but within a few months I was called in by the bosses to be told that *GMTV* was considering setting up a permanent bureau in Los Angeles – and they wanted me to run it! It would mean packing up and moving to the United States, finding an office, getting it established and then recording reports for the show twice a week. The best thing about it was I would be working permanently with Neal.

I was thrilled. What an adventure!

Los Angeles was a good life. To begin with, I lived in a flat while I found something more permanent. I was spending every waking hour building contacts and sending my twice-weekly reports about Hollywood life back to London. But I was fast asleep in January 1994 when the biggest story in years happened – the Northridge earthquake that devastated the Los Angeles area. I was sleeping on a mattress on the floor as I hadn't even bought a bed by that point when I felt something strange going on. I couldn't work out what it was, but I felt entirely disorientated. The next thing I knew someone was banging on the front door of the flat. When I went to open it, there was Neal, looking slightly dishevelled and very frantic.

'There's been an earthquake,' he said. 'Get your stuff together, we need to get to the centre of it all and start reporting.'

A horrendous shock had hit the city – fifty-seven people had been killed and thousands injured – but somehow I'd managed to sleep through the whole thing.

We jumped straight in the car and I drove into the city centre. Fires had broken out on both sides of the road as the electricity and gas had gone down. There were gaping chasms in some of the roads too. I was terrified another one could emerge right in front of us on the highway, but there was no question of not going to the centre of the 'quake – we had to make sure we were there to send reports of the chaos back to London as soon as *GMTV* came on air.

It was such a sad story because so many people had been killed, injured or forced to leave their homes, but it was also incredibly exciting to be on the scene for such a massive news event. There was no doubt in my mind this was the job I had been working towards all my life.

After a few months, I found myself a sweet little wooden house – more of a shack really – on the outskirts of LA. Surrounded by trees, it even had a friendly skunk living in the backyard. It was quite secluded, considering it was in one of the busiest places on earth, and so pretty, like *Little House on the Prairie* next to the city.

'Are you sure you're going to be OK here?' Neal asked as I proudly showed him around my new home.

'What do you mean?' I replied.

'Well, it's like something from the backwoods. Aren't you worried you'll be all alone in the middle of the night, surrounded by trees?'

'Don't be daft,' I said, my independence flaring to the surface. 'Of course not.'

And I wasn't. Living in my own little home, reporting on Hollywood and coming up with my own story ideas each day was the independence and excitement I adored. I never felt scared or alone. People made too much fuss about things that could go wrong when usually things went pretty well. And I loved having a sanctuary to come back to at the end of a hectic day at work. I'd found myself a little Mazda MX-5 convertible so was whizzing around Los Angeles from job to job – it really was living the dream. But I never fell for the Hollywood hype. I was there to do a job, not to try to get myself a part in the next Bruce Willis blockbuster.

Neal and I kept our feet firmly on the ground. We were hanging out together most weekends and evenings, often with other Brit journalists based in the city too. We spent our evenings at different restaurants and bars then at weekends, we would often zip off to Pasadena, further down the valley in California. We'd go for walks, do a bit of shopping and have dinner, and generally just enjoy the more laid-back lifestyle.

When we first met, we had both come out of relationships and were feeling a bit raw so we supported each other through that. There was never any question that we would be more than friends. Together we could laugh at our disasters while feeling safe in the knowledge that we'd each found a friend who would be there for the other.

Our second Oscars was much more of a success. This time we found the perfect spot on the red carpet and bagged every celebrity coming out of the ceremony. I talked to Steven Spielberg, whose epic drama *Schindler's List* had just won seven Oscars. He was lovely. And then Leonardo DiCaprio was so funny, leaping around all over the place. He was still a baby-faced nineteen-year-old who had been nominated as Best Supporting Actor for his role in the coming-of-age film *What's Eating Gilbert Grape*. He was absolutely adorable.

And then we chatted to Ralph Fiennes, who had been nominated for Best Supporting Actor for his role in *Schindler's List*.

A couple of weeks earlier, Neal and I had bumped into Ralph in a cafe and he was always happy to chat whenever I'd run up to him and say hi.

'Don't forget to come over and chat to us on the red carpet!' I laughed.

'Of course I will,' he replied.

And he did.

When I saw Emma Thompson (nominee for both Best Actress and Best Supporting Actress) getting into her chauffeur-driven car further down the road I went sprinting down there in my high heels, trying to get her to chat to us before she left. But too late – the car sped off, leaving me out of breath and out of luck.

I ran back again to our spot on the carpet, crammed in alongside reporters and camera crews from around the world, and managed to get a brilliant interview with Anthony Hopkins, who had been nominated as Best Actor for *The Remains of the Day*. He was such a lovely man. So charming.

All in all, it was a hugely successful night. We left no stone unturned so people back home in Britain got a little taste of what it was like to be at the biggest showbiz night of the year. I could be quite sharp-elbowed when I needed to be, but it worked. And the bosses in London seemed delighted with what Neal and I were achieving.

When we were out on jobs, Neal could get a bit stressed about how on earth we were going to nail a particularly tricky interview. Or he would be constantly dragging on a cigarette, coming up with more and more ideas of stories we could try.

I was a bit more relaxed and knew we would make whatever we wanted to do work. What was exactly the same about us though was that we were both hungry for exclusives and stories that would be leading the news back in Britain.

In truth, both Neal and I were more than a bit obsessed with work – we were a reporting team match made in heaven. We didn't just want to be padding the show with light showbiz fluff. I was up for everything and wanted to do the very best I could in LA and never give anyone back in London the excuse to say I wasn't giving this incredible opportunity my very best shot. We were the only British broadcast team in town, which helped enormously in landing interviews. The BBC and others were all based in Washington or New York – the 'serious' side of the United States.

The biggest story we covered while I was there was, without doubt, the Michael Jackson scandal, which first broke in 1993. I had been around at Neal's apartment and, completely by chance, we were watching the news in the middle of the after-noon when a reporter popped up saying: 'We are receiving news that police officers are quizzing Michael Jackson over allegations made against him. We are waiting for more infor-mation as to what this is all about.'

Neal and I had no idea either, but I was certain of one thing: 'This is big,' I told him. 'We need to find out what's going on.'

About ten minutes later Michael Jackson's lawyer gave a statement saying: 'This has absolutely nothing to do with child abuse.'

At which point I said: 'This isn't big, this is absolutely massive.'

Within minutes we were up and running. That night, the Los Angeles Police Department said they would be making a statement shortly. But that meant it would be after *GMTV* went off air, which was no good for me.

'Please,' I said to the LAPD press officer who I was dealing with. 'Please can you give us an early look at the statement. We are working to London time and this is a huge story.'

And they gave us the statement – a world exclusive on the inquiry into Michael Jackson. That was so LA though! Nowhere else in the world would a police department work around filming schedules.

Three days later I spotted that the Jackson family were doing a press interview about a project they were trying to promote (nothing to do with Michael!). The only reporter allowed in was a very serious one from Reuters, but I managed to somehow talk my way into the room too. There was a massive intake of breath when I said: 'So what about these allegations about Michael then? Are the allegations true?'

It was the question they were totally trying to avoid – but the question that the rest of the world wanted answered.

We packed so much into the three years I was in LA. One day Phil Collins' ex-wife got in touch because she wanted to open her heart about what had gone wrong in their marriage. Then the next week I was interviewing Liberace in his incredible over-the-top mansion. I chatted to Jane Seymour on the set of *Dr Quinn, Medicine Woman* and to Mickey Rourke in his gym. He was so honest and raw, it was incredible.

One of my favourites was the singer Donny Osmond. We got on so well and kept in touch afterwards. So much so that years later after I was married, Martin was leaving his office in London one day when a guy called over to him: 'Hey, you're Martin. You're married to Fiona Phillips – I love Fiona.'

It was Donny!

Poor Martin. He'd already lost his first-ever girlfriend to her devotion to Donny – he didn't want me going the same way!

On another assignment we reported from the beach where Dudley Moore was getting married. And before the ceremony he even came over for a long chat. The O. J. Simpson case was rumbling on during that period too so there was always news to report.

We even flew over to New York for a live *GMTV* show, which I presented with Eamonn Holmes from near Times Square with Eartha Kitt on the sofa! That was the first time I'd met Eamonn – he was very friendly and a great professional. I didn't realize then we would soon be together almost every single day.

But despite the excitement of life in LA, I always kept in touch with home, ringing Mum at least once a week. If Dad ever answered, he would say, 'Oh, hello. What's it like out there then?' Then it would be, 'I'll get your mum.' That was it – he never enjoyed talking on the telephone.

And I realized my life was a long way from his in so many ways. I wonder now how he must have felt about all this. He never said so, but I think, like Mum, he was proud of me. But for a man who had seen so many of his dreams come to nothing, I wonder if it hurt to see how, unlike for him, life had worked out pretty well for his only daughter. Now I hope he understood it was his work ethic that had got me there. That and his stubbornness.

My brother David came out for a visit and then I persuaded Mum and Dad to visit too. I knew I wanted to return to London at some point to do more presenting and it was important to me that my parents saw my LA life before it was too late. It was a big thing for them to travel all the way to the West Coast of America, though, but after months and months of persuasion they agreed. Unfortunately, it wasn't the dream reunion I'd hoped for. Without us having any awareness, something new and corrosive had joined our family: Alzheimer's.

Nothing would ever be the same again.

I'll tell you about that trip later. For now, I just want to focus on the good times of those years in LA. One of the best was in my final months in Hollywood when we reported on the 1996 Oscars ceremony. It was the year *Braveheart* won five Oscars, including Best Movie and Best Director for Mel Gibson. After the ceremony he must have been on cloud nine but he came down the red carpet and headed straight for Neal and me. We had such a laugh together and he even let me hold his two Oscar trophies to check how heavy they were!

The bosses in London must have thought that I'd been doing a good job because over the past year or so they had been calling me back to stand in whenever the main *GMTV* presenter – Anthea Turner – went on holiday. That meant 3.30 a.m. starts to be in the studio in time to get on top of the morning's news, prep for interviews, get hair and make-up done and rehearse any tricky bits of the show. I was always sat alongside Eamonn Holmes, who worked hard to make me feel comfortable in the role, although there was little doubt who was in charge. And God forbid I should want to take the lead in interviewing a politician or anyone 'serious'. In that, I was very much in a supporting role!

Covering for Anthea meant quite a bit of flying backwards and forwards to LA but it was a great opportunity to anchor the show and I was very conscious that I had a lot to learn. Eamonn definitely helped me with that.

By 1996, I was ready to return home permanently. I had loved LA but I was keen to go back to reporting in the UK and it felt like there would be more opportunities for presenting in London too. It was time to go home. I told Neal, who had also been looking for a change. It was the end of our glorious adventure Stateside.

As I've been talking and writing all this about our hilarious Hollywood escapades, Neal has been sat with me. He lives in Bali on the other side of the world now so we only occasionally see each other. It feels very special that he is here in London as I try to remember the times we had together. Going through his incredible collection of old pictures, which have jogged my memory, we have laughed about the ridiculous stunts we got up to. And we have cried too about how long ago that carefree existence seems to be. Sometimes Neal cries too and I wonder if his tears are for me or for the Fiona he used to know.

7

I hope this book isn't going backwards and forwards too much in my memories for you to keep up. If so, sorry, but welcome to my world! One minute I'm remembering every detail of the first evening I went for dinner with Martin (with Neal in tow, of course!) and then I'm struggling to remember where I keep the coffee cups in my own kitchen. I'm remembering and forgetting all the emotional things too. The way I felt about Martin, when we got together properly and that wild excitement of falling in love. Sometimes it's a distant memory compared to how I feel now, when I know I'm withdrawn or not always easy to live with.

So let's go back a bit to meeting Martin.

I was due to return home for a stint in December 1995 to cover Anthea Turner's Christmas holiday. *GMTV* were sending out another reporter, Martin Frizell, to cover for me. There would be just one evening crossover between our flights in and out of Los Angeles – long enough for me to fill him in on any events or issues he needed to know about.

How one evening can stretch to three decades!

I'd met Martin three years earlier, when he was a reporter at Sky, and again when he became chief correspondent of *GMTV*, but only really to say hello. To be honest, I'd always thought he took himself a bit too seriously. He seemed a slightly aloof, arrogant Scotsman who was rather pleased with himself. Goodness knows what he thought about me when I was a reporter. Probably that I was difficult and always going around moaning about how I'd been passed over for the best stories!

Still, Neal and I thought we owed Martin dinner when he arrived in LA to ensure he had a proper handover before I went back to England. When we met at the restaurant I still hadn't packed, wrapped any Christmas presents for Mum and Dad or even tidied my house, and I was going to have to be up at the crack of dawn to catch the flight. I really could have done without having to go out that evening, but actually it was fine. OK, it was better than fine. It was lovely. *He* was lovely.

Martin wasn't arrogant or cocky at all – he was asking for advice on who to go to for help on certain stories and seemed quite nervous about the scale of reporting from Hollywood. In fact, I found him quite vulnerable and uncertain of himself. Not so uncertain that he didn't ask if he could come back to mine for coffee afterwards though!

'Er, no, I don't think so,' I said firmly.

It was about five hours until my flight by then. Any 'coffee dates' would have to wait.

By the summer of 1996, I was back working in London. I saw Martin around the *GMTV* offices and we chatted, but

I wasn't sure that things would develop. Anyway, I was busy getting back into life in Britain, catching up with friends and spending as much time as I could in Wales with Mum and Dad. Then in June, he and I were sent with a full crew to do a live show from the races at Ascot. I was anchoring the show and Martin was to go out and about around the racecourse reporting.

We all bundled onto a minibus at 3 a.m. for the drive down to Ascot. It was a glorious summer's morning and one of those days when you have to pinch yourself: *Seriously, am I being paid for this? To appear on live television at one of the most prestigious events in the national calendar?* Don't get me wrong, it was hard work making everything run smoothly for the viewers at home when there was almost always some disaster just moments away. But how lucky was I to be doing it?

The show was over by nine and then after a bit of time in Ascot we all trooped back onto the bus and were back at the *GMTV* studios by noon. Martin and I had been chatting (OK, flirting) on the bus back to London.

'So do you fancy a bit of lunch?' he asked.

The sun was shining and we'd already done a day's work, so why not?

We went to a little Italian restaurant that I knew, which was very relaxed and they didn't mind if you sat there all afternoon drinking wine. Just as well. We stayed there for hours, drinking and sharing the stories of our lives. Martin had journalism in his veins – his dad had been sports editor of the *News of the World*'s Scottish edition – and Martin had worked his way up from a local newspaper to reporting for Radio Clyde before coming to London. He was very focused and had an incredible work ethic. Obviously, I found that very attractive – and other stuff too!

It was mid-evening before we left, knowing we'd have to be up again at 3.30 a.m. to get back on shift. We walked from the restaurant towards his flat. When we got there, I kissed him on the cheek, then carried on walking the ten minutes back home.

I wasn't going to let him get everything he wanted too soon! But I think we both knew that day we were already in deep. This was something special and soon we were spending every spare hour we had together. We tried to keep our relationship quiet at work as I didn't want us to become the new *GMTV* gossip, but I think some people must have guessed – we were both a little obsessed with each other.

And then, four weeks after that first afternoon, after another long summer lunch, Martin dropped what felt like an emotional nuclear bomb.

'Er, would you think about marrying me?' he said.

'What?' I gasped.

'Yeah, would you . . .?'

I was stunned. Absolutely floored. I knew things had been moving fast and we had completely fallen for each other, but marriage . . . That still felt like the sort of thing other people did. Not me. And, to be honest, I wasn't entirely convinced it was a good idea. When Dad had told me: 'Don't ever get married,' I'd thought it was pretty good advice. Everything I'd worked for and achieved up until that point had been to give myself independence. Every relationship I'd had, however good it had been, had ended up hitting the rocks when I began to feel suffocated and a need for freedom – the thought of marriage made me gasp for breath.

'Oh, I don't think I'm suited to marriage,' I told Martin. 'I'm just not good at being tied down.'

And that was me back then – utterly, entirely independent. Thank God I had no idea how much that would change in the years to come or what a gift independence is for the young and healthy.

I'm not sure if Martin had thought through what my response to a marriage proposal would be but clearly he hadn't expected that. I watched in horror as his eyes filled with tears. Still a proud man, he turned his head away.

'I didn't think I would ever want to marry either,' he conceded. 'But now I do.'

There was no gushing romance or over-emotional protestations, just Martin's usual clear focused approach to life. Here was a situation where he wanted something and he was going to do whatever he could to get it, like landing a great scoop or pulling off an interview. I could see how the idea of marriage struck him as the most logical thing in the world in the situation he'd found himself in and I was starting to wonder if maybe I did too. What I definitely did *not* want was the big meringue dress, a troupe of bridesmaids or a bouquet stretching to the ground. Yes, that had always been Mum's dream for me, but the whole thing made me feel queasy. So I never gave him an outright 'no' and gradually the idea seemed less and less shocking to me.

There was no doubt I was in love with Martin and wanted to be with him. But marriage? Maybe there was some kind of compromise we could find.

Even the thought of moving out of my lovely little flat and into Martin's place in south-west London seemed at first like a leap, but we were spending almost every night together anyway so it was the logical thing to do. And it worked because Martin was his own man. He never smothered me, but he was always there to support me when I needed it. And he was no pushover either. I admired that. Most importantly, we had fun together.

That year, Anthea Turner decided to quit *GMTV*. There had been rumours in the press – not to mention the newsroom – for ages that she and fellow presenter Eamonn Holmes weren't getting on at all well and she'd had enough. Eamonn thought Anthea was vain and called her 'Princess Tippy Toes', which ended up in the press. Meanwhile Anthea was the latest victim of the sexist world of TV in those days where men were allowed to be ambitious and outspoken, but when women behaved that way they were deemed to be pushy.

With Anthea gone, there was a vacancy for her job on the sofa. I was called in to cover for her while they came up with a full-time replacement. Obviously, I was hopeful they might choose me and I worked hard to do my very best so they might, but there were some other strong contenders in the frame.

The gossipmongers and newspaper showbiz reporters went into overdrive about who would get the role. There were endless stories about who it would be and all the leaks from *GMTV* indicated that the job would go to presenter Ulrika Jonsson. It reached the point where I sort of accepted that while the powers that be were happy for me to stand in when they needed me, maybe they didn't want me in the job full-time. Martin and I decided to get away from it all with a holiday to the Isle of Mull. He had always loved the west coast of Scotland and wanted to introduce me to its wild scenery. We had such a lovely time, going for walks along the beach and spending cosy evenings in local pubs. I'd almost managed to forget the hullabaloo of who would get the *GMTV* job when my phone rang one afternoon: it was the office. They wanted me to go back to London for a conversation.

A conversation about me becoming the new host of *GMTV*.

I was thrilled. Utterly delighted. I felt like the luckiest woman in the world. And not only did I secure the job of my dreams, I was in love with a man who accepted me just the way I was. Martin didn't want to change me or clip my wings, he wanted to support me.

Maybe Dad had been entirely wrong about marriage.

And gradually the idea of marriage grew, but it would be on our terms.

'Let's go to Las Vegas!' I suggested to Martin one day late in 1996.

He was up for it. We knew we would have to break it to our parents when we got home and they might not be best pleased, but we also knew they would understand – the whole big wedding thing wasn't really suited to either of us.

We had just booked flights, though, when Dad called with terrible news: Mum had been diagnosed with breast cancer.

For a while, the wedding was on hold. But, as the weeks passed, Martin and I became increasingly certain that it was what we wanted to do. We wanted that sense of absolute commitment, even if we didn't want the three tiers of wedding cake and the bouquet of pink lilies that were fashionable in those days. We rebooked our flights for Las Vegas and flew out without telling anyone. Martin had booked a room at the luxurious Caesars Palace and then, on 7 May 1997, we were married at the Little Chapel of the Flowers. Our limo chauffeur, whom we'd never seen before in our lives until that day, was our only witness. And it was amazing!

Martin was in a black suit and I wore a black floor-length dress, which he'd bought me. It was the marriage we wanted in the way we wanted it. It was perfect. I loved Martin so much and now we were a team – I could be myself but feel utterly secure. Afterwards the limo driver took pictures of us outside the chapel and then the two of us went for a Chinese meal before wandering down the Strip, playing on some of the slot machines. It couldn't have been more low-key, but it was marriage, something I'd said I'd never do. How would I tell Dad? But actually, it felt OK.

The next day we drove to Santa Monica for our honeymoon. It was bliss. We stayed at the very swanky Shutters on the Beach hotel. So swanky that when we were walking through the lobby I heard a strong Mancunian voice shouting, 'Oi, Phillips! What are you doing here?'

Martin and I turned to see Liam and Noel Gallagher of Oasis in the lounge with two very attractive young women – who I don't think were their partners at the time! I'd interviewed Liam a few times and he was always lovely. A few years later, when he split from his wife Patsy Kensit, he insisted I was the only reporter he wanted to talk to about it. I don't know why – maybe he liked watching *GMTV* while he ate his cornflakes. That evening was funny though.

Noel said: 'If anyone asks, you didn't see us!'

Martin and I went on enjoying our honeymoon, our marriage a wonderful secret from the rest of the world. Except a week later we were back in London. And back to reality.

A reality that was increasingly painful.

8

The sinister part of Alzheimer's disease is that it takes root in your mind without you even knowing it. It has started its terrible work before you even feel a bit 'not quite yourself' and by the time it becomes apparent to those closest to you, it is well into establishing itself, like one of those ivy plants that binds itself to a tree and becomes impossible to dig out.

That's definitely how it was with Mum. When I think back, there were lots of times we thought she was being a bit crazy or ditzy over the years. But that was Mum. Where did her naturally bubbly but sometimes scatty behaviour end and Alzheimer's begin? I'm really not sure.

Even before I went out to work in LA – when Mum would have still been in only her mid-fifties – there were things that seemed unusual, but never for one moment did I imagine she was facing the beginning of Alzheimer's. She was living in Wales with Dad and Andrew then and while I would pop down for weekends and holidays, maybe I missed some changes in her personality because I wasn't there all the time. She had always suffered with headaches and what I realize now was probably clinical depression. And it did feel as if her spells of depression were becoming more frequent, but she was a woman in her fifties and, back then, it was often just quietly assumed that 'women of a certain age' would 'live on their nerves', as Mum herself would say.

I remember when I was a reporter in London, long before I met Martin, I took a new boyfriend to Wales with me to visit Mum and Dad. He got on brilliantly with Dad, going for a pint down the local pub with him, but he thought Mum was a bit 'reserved' and 'offish'. No one would ever have said that about Mum years earlier. She was the warmest person you could imagine. She was the only woman I knew who could nip out for a pint of milk then not return for three hours because she'd found so many people to talk to.

Why had she become so introverted?

Then there was the day of a cousin's wedding in Cambridge, soon after I started work at *GMTV*. For weeks, Mum had been excited about it – she had got her new outfit and a hat from Marks & Spencer and was so looking forward to seeing the family. But, in the final few days before the wedding, she became really stressed about the whole thing. By the time we arrived in Cambridge, she was totally out of sorts. She seemed kind of brittle, like she might collapse in tears at any moment, and then kept disappearing off to the loo every ten minutes.

'You OK, Mum?' I asked a couple of times, but that only seemed to irritate her and she quickly nodded.

I should have insisted she tell me what was really going on, but it didn't seem the moment and we had been used to Mum having her bad patches all our lives – it seemed to be just another one of those. But during the reception it got so much worse. After the best man's speech, Mum stood up for the toast and her skirt fell down (she must have been to the loo and forgotten to zip it up). She hadn't been drinking so it wasn't a case of one glass of bubbly too many. Everyone laughed and Dad joked about it, but Mum looked mortified.

I was standing there with my new boyfriend and felt totally embarrassed – embarrassed for Mum but, I'm ashamed to say, I was embarrassed for myself too.

What was wrong with her?

Which was what she asked me when I found her later on crying in the toilets of the hotel, where the reception was being held.

'I don't know what's wrong with me,' she said.

'You're probably just a bit rundown,' I replied in that way people try to comfort others without offering any actual comfort at all.

Mum had been to her GP in Wales, who concluded she was struggling with the menopause and put her on hormone replacement therapy. He'd said it would ease her feelings of anxiety and depression. It wasn't making much difference though. And when Mum and Dad went home after the wedding, it just got worse.

When I'd ring her from work, she'd be distant or weepy. I didn't understand what was happening either and it was frustrating – I wanted my mum back. If only I could have been a bit more sympathetic.

I know I talk a lot about my mum now and what it was like to watch her terrifying descent into Alzheimer's. I'm also aware I did a lot of newspaper interviews about her when she became more seriously ill, but I feel I couldn't write this book now without telling the whole story again. Because so often it feels like Mum's and my stories are entirely interwoven. Not only did I most likely get this terrible illness in some way from my parents, but the way that depression and anxiety ushered it in also seems similar and of course I witnessed it all as it progressed. Like watching a trailer for my own life with Alzheimer's. Thank God I didn't realize it at the time – that would have been too much to manage.

Sometimes, though, Mum would seem like her old self and I'd put my worries that she was becoming ill out of my mind for a couple of months. Now I wonder if that was her putting on a brave face for me on those calls or whether there were days when she could pull free from the cloud enfolding her. She must have been sufficiently concerned to chat to friends about what was happening. Goodness knows who, but one of them must have suggested she try Transcendental Meditation (or 'Incidental Medication' as she called it). She would try to sit in the chair and meditate, which apparently was going to stop her mind getting clogged up with the worries of everyday life.

Of course it didn't make any difference.

When I did get home for a weekend, Mum would be there fussing over me, cooking tea, doing my washing and being just like Mum, chatting on and on while Dad stayed glued to the telly. She would sometimes flit from subject to subject or occasionally get her words muddled up or forget halfway through a sentence what she was meaning to tell us, but that was just my bubbly, scatty mum. Or at least that's what I thought.

She loved getting the coach up from Wales to visit me in London. You could guarantee she'd get off the coach at Victoria bus station accompanied by the person she'd been sat next to for the entire trip. She would know their life story inside out, having plied them with Welsh cakes and her own stories about her oh-so-successful daughter and her handsome sons, David and Andrew.

We'd have the best weekends together, shopping or going for walks, taking in the sights. They were probably the times I felt closest to Mum. It feels particularly sad now that we had the time to talk then but so much remained unspoken between us. There were little things that increasingly bothered me about Mum's behaviour – and must have worried her too – but none of them on their own seemed particularly serious. I knew she had become anxious about working on the tills at the department store where she'd been employed for years. But Mum had never been great at new technology – even the idea of operating a new washing machine would put her into a spin.

Then there was the time she got in a muddle with her Abbey National cashpoint card and the building society staff had to help her work it. But once again, I rationalized it – Mum had never liked all these 'modern machines' and much preferred a smartly dressed man in the bank, with whom she could have a proper chat, than a hole in the wall.

For every incident that seemed a little odd there was always an explanation. I guess the mistake we all made was looking at those incidents in isolation – we never joined the dots to make sense of what was really going on with Mum.

At times I did think there was something 'bigger' going on and I worried that my parents' always difficult marriage might be in the process of totally collapsing. Again, we didn't discuss it as a family as we should have done but I thought that was perhaps the cause of Mum's spells of weepiness. Dad had lost his managerial job at the TV rental company and felt more than ever that the world was against him. Now in his early sixties, he was back scraping a living from repairing TVs – the job he'd started out doing more than thirty years earlier. His frustrated dreams and anger at the world seemed to bubble beneath the surface of his every conversation. It never occurred to him that his ability to fall out with people might be the cause of his problems. Mum's increased ditziness or days of weeping made him furious – it was like everything in his work, life and marriage had amounted to nothing.

One day, things totally exploded at home. I wasn't there, but Mum told me the whole story on the phone later. She and Dad had been bickering pretty much as they always did, when Dad totally flipped. He grabbed Mum around the neck and almost throttled her. My little brother Andrew, who was still only seventeen, saw the whole thing. Then Dad turned on him and grabbed him around the neck too. It was the final straw for Andrew. He'd been the only child trapped inside Mum and Dad's battlefield marriage ever since they moved back to Wales.

He chucked some clothes and books in a black bin bag and moved into a friend's house.

Mum was devastated.

Devastated that her husband had turned on her and on her adored baby son, but also that between them they'd now forced Andrew out of the family home. Mum begged Andrew to come back, but he point-blank refused.

Now I'm not making excuses for my dad one bit. What he did was entirely wrong, but sometimes I wonder if having to cope with Mum's erratic behaviour for so long without understanding the causes behind it had made him deeply frustrated. On top of that, he was having to deal with his own life's disappointments.

The whole thing was a mess.

Mum was broken for weeks after that. When David and I met her at Victoria bus station on her next visit up to London shortly before I moved to LA, she got off the coach and broke down in tears. But still I thought she was just sad that our family was falling apart. If only I'd taken the time to try to find out what was really going on – how she must have been feeling increasingly unanchored and confused. There's so much I understand all too well now, but at the time I really couldn't see.

Like I said earlier, Mum and Dad came to visit me in June 1994 when I was living in Los Angeles and that was when I really noticed a change in her. Neal came with me to collect my parents from the airport and, within minutes, I was tearing my hair out. They were tired and grumpy and I felt like they were trying to blame me for dragging them so far from home. It all just seemed a bit much for them – Mum couldn't even work out how to get down the escalator.

'Maybe they're just too old for this,' I said to Neal.

Although, looking back, they were still only in their early sixties.

What I hadn't considered was that Mum hadn't even been on an aeroplane before and Dad's globe-trotting days in the Royal Navy were a long way behind him by then. For years they had been living a very quiet life in west Wales. But there was something else not right too. Mum was so nervy and anxious; she'd have bursts of chattiness and bubbliness, but it seemed they took up a huge amount of her energy. Even when we'd got back to the cosy hotel I'd booked for them and set them up with a proper cup of English tea, things still weren't quite 'right' – it seemed like the two of them were barely speaking to each other.

One afternoon during their trip we went out for coffee and again, Mum was distant and teary. I felt hurt and angry. I'd so hoped that they would have the trip of a lifetime and enjoy spending time with me, but I couldn't have been more wrong.

'I don't know why you bothered to come if you're going to be like this,' I snapped. 'I can't believe you're in this incredible place and you're being so miserable.'

Dad looked at Mum more softly than he ever usually did, but he didn't say anything more. Neither did she. Or me. Whatever was going on remained unsaid.

I was partly relieved, partly cross with them for their behaviour and partly consumed with guilt that I had snapped at them when Mum was clearly struggling. But why couldn't they enjoy spending time with me? Why did everything always have to be so complicated?

I kept up to date with things at home through my weekly phone calls from Mum. Whenever I returned from LA to cover for Anthea Turner, I would visit as often as I could. I got the impression things still weren't great between her and Dad. They rarely went out together and never went on holiday again after that dismal trip to LA. Dad was back working every hour he could. I don't know whether it was because he desperately needed the money, was still driven by his work ethic or maybe, and this is the bit that makes me sad, he just no longer wanted to be at home with Mum. There was a general sense around him that his whole life had been a failure: 'So it's come to this, then?' he'd say, shaking his head. He had lost all interest and patience with Mum entirely.

It had never been the love affair of the century, but now they were living entirely separate lives. Mum appeared heartbroken. All those years where she had hero-worshipped him and now he simply found her an annoyance. In hindsight, I think they were both suffering from extreme depression. Mum would cry and Dad would huff about 'that bloody woman' and walk out of the room. But at the time I didn't really understand depression – I just thought they were being Mum and Dad, but more so than ever before.

Dad rarely spoke to me on the phone – I think dads rarely

do – so I had no idea if he was aware that Mum's behaviour was becoming more erratic. When I saw her, she could sometimes behave oddly, but this had been going on for so long by then it was hard to remember what was normal.

Things deteriorated even further when Martin made the pilgrimage west to meet Mum and Dad for the first time, in the autumn of 1996. I was on tenterhooks because I knew how unpredictable Mum's behaviour could be, but at the same time I desperately wanted everyone to get on. Sure enough, though, after I'd picked up Martin from the station and collected Mum from work at the department store, she barely spoke to him – it was so rude. But Mum seemed to have no interest in this new man in her daughter's life. Years before she would have known his entire life story before he was on his second cup of tea.

Later that evening, Mum cheered up a bit and took pictures of us sitting on the sofa. I was mortified, with my head in my hands. Years later, I found a photo with her notes on the back. She'd written: 'Fiona was annoyed at me takein pictures'. Her handwriting was messy and slipped between capitals and lowercase and she has totally misspelt 'taking'. When I was growing up, her spelling had been impeccable.

Soon after, Mum and Dad came up to London for David's wedding to his long-term girlfriend, Sarah. It was so lovely to see David so happy, but Mum and Dad turned up with no sense of excitement at all. As ever, they were irritable and snapping at each other. Despite still only being in their mid-sixties, they looked so old. Andrew, David and I would chat about how tired

Mum and Dad were looking, but we had been used to their difficult marriage for years. We didn't think this was anything more serious than that.

A couple of weeks after the wedding we found out why Mum had been looking particularly frail. When my mobile rang and it was Dad I knew it had to be bad news. I don't think he'd ever rung me before – and definitely not on my mobile!

Calls home were always Mum and me, then right at the end her saying, 'I'll put your dad on the phone.' At best, there would be a one-minute exchange along the lines of 'How's work going?', but phone calls just weren't something he did. This time, he got straight to the point: 'It's your mum,' he said. 'The doctors say she has breast cancer.'

I felt a bit sick. No wonder she'd looked so pale and unwell at David's wedding. It later turned out she had known all through the wedding about the cancer but hadn't wanted to tell anyone. She'd only got herself tested because there was one of those mobile screening vans parked up outside Tesco when she'd been doing her weekly shop. Now the fear was that not only did she need a mastectomy, but also that the disease might have spread to her bones.

The mastectomy was booked for Christmas Eve 1996, which meant us kids spent Christmas Day around her hospital bed trying to bring a bit of festive cheer. It was tough. Mum was tired and even when she shone that dazzling smile towards us, I could tell it was just for show, to remind us how she used to be. It felt like someone had switched off a light inside her.

David told me later that she'd said to him: 'I'm ready to go now, Day.'

How had she lost all pleasure in life?

Martin was brilliant during this time and joined me on the regular trips up and down the M4 as I kept checking up on her recovery. Even when she seemed physically better, emotionally, she remained very flat. The whole house looked as if it could do with a good clean. Mum had always been so house-proud, but now there were kitchen dishes left lying on the side overnight and there was never much in the fridge to eat. At the time, I thought it was Mum and Dad just giving up on operating like a couple and each doing their own thing.

I still thought maybe menopause was the problem, but I was convinced the hormone replacement therapy the doctor had put Mum on in her mid-fifties was what had caused her breast cancer. There were a lot of reports at that time linking HRT and breast cancer. And then after her surgery she was to be on a five-year prescription of Tamoxifen, another hormone therapy drug for breast cancer. I'd always hated the idea of any synthetic medication – it can't be right stuffing your body with all those chemicals. More recently, expert research has shown that I shouldn't have been concerned – but back then I was.

All this was still in the early days of my relationship with Martin, even though we were planning to marry. Goodness knows what he must have thought about my crazy family. He was so patient. There was the excruciating time Dad started yelling at Mum in a restaurant as she cried, all because she wanted the portable telly moved into her bedroom. And the time I invited Mum to join us at Crufts dog show in Birmingham and she got entirely lost getting from the train station to the hotel. All my stories about Mum were of this warm, wonderful, bubbly woman who loved cooking for her family and fussing over them, but all Martin was seeing was a withdrawn woman who barely took an interest in her children's lives and had mood swings, going from being outgoing one day to absolute silence the next.

There were times I wondered if Mum didn't like Martin – she was so disinterested in either of us when we went to visit. But I don't think it was that. And he was so kind and considerate of her – 'a well-brought-up young man' she might have said years earlier.

I think having all that confusion going on in my family was another reason I wanted to disappear off to Vegas for our wedding. I knew Mum and Dad hadn't really enjoyed David's wedding. Dad hated all that getting dressed up and making small talk with relatives he hadn't seen for years or strangers he'd never met at all. And even though Mum had dreamed for years I'd have a big white wedding one day like all her friends' daughters, by then she'd given up on that hope.

And it felt like even a wedding wouldn't cheer up Mum nowadays.

At least if Martin and I were married in Vegas, one thing I wouldn't be worrying about for once was my parents.

When Martin and I flew back to London after our wedding in May 1997, I immediately rang my parents to say their oh-so-independent daughter had finally got hitched. Despite

Dad's years of persuading me not to marry, he was pleased for us. He liked Martin and knew he was a good man. Mum was fairly disinterested. She didn't even ask what I'd worn, which would always have been her number-one question.

'Auntie Mary always said you'd run off and get married,' she told me.

I had to accept that she might be cross that I'd deprived her of her big Mother of the Bride moment, but it was more than that – it was like she didn't even really care. And that hurt.

9

Although my memories of life are becoming reduced, many of those that remain are about Mum. And particularly about the period of her illness and decline.

I talk about it a lot. Is that because I feel guilty that I wasn't able to do more to help her and that she had to go into a care home? Or maybe it sits with me so much because it was all so horribly traumatic.

I hope I've painted a good picture for you of what Mum was like when my brothers and I were little. She was an amazing woman – the kindest, warmest, most loving mum anyone could hope to have. But she suffered so much sadness. My over-whelming sense when I think of her now is one of sorrow. She suffered so much with depression, which slipped into her agonizing, bewildering experience with Alzheimer's.

I tried so hard to look after her and bring some happiness in her final years, but I remain overwhelmed with guilt that there wasn't more I could do. Maybe it still looms large for me because deep down, there was always a fear that I might be watching my own future play out in front of me. I don't really think it was that, though – mainly it was just heartachingly sad to see the woman who had done everything for me being taken away, moment by moment. And the fear she had of not knowing what was happening to her.

Utter, utter fear.

And I wasn't able to prevent that.

All that work, all those hours of trying to be successful and the perfect daughter she could be proud of, but when it came to it I wasn't good enough to save her. That's what lingers with me. And that's the cruelty of Alzheimer's. Not just for those 'living with it' but for all those around them desperately trying to ease their pain, but being entirely incapable of doing so.

The next chapter of my memories talks about those early years of my life as a new mum. I loved the time I spent with my baby boys so much, even though I was combining my role as a new mother with the early starts of breakfast TV. And yet whatever was going on during that time, Mum was always with me in my mind – the worry of Mum and how she was suffering never left me.

Alzheimer's is like that – the fear, frustration and confusion of it sucks in everyone around, even if they're hundreds of miles away. Let me explain . . .

10

It was early in 1997 when I took my seat permanently on the famous *GMTV* sofa alongside Eamonn Holmes. I was thrilled to have the job, although equally terrified – I couldn't quite believe it was going to be me beaming into people's front rooms all over Britain every morning.

The job was tough – it meant 3.30 a.m. starts each day so no late nights out partying. There was no way you could do that job without being totally alert. Every morning there was news breaking, directions being barked down my earpiece, guests going missing and all sorts of chaos, but I just had to keep on smiling and make it all look entirely effortless.

I loved it. And I loved the life Martin and I were building together. We had bought a lovely little house in south London, which we spent our weekends decorating and turning into a home. Other times we would enjoy long, leisurely lunches then trail around local shops looking for bits and bobs for the house. We visited Martin's family in Scotland and went back and forth to Wales a lot as well – I was constantly anxious about things at home.

Mum would still get the coach up to visit. She seemed to enjoy that. Martin and I had some lovely holidays too. We were both working and, with no children of our own, we decided to enjoy ourselves.

In the summer of 1998 we had an incredible trip to Barbados. A couple of weeks later, I discovered I was pregnant.

As you might have realized by now, I've never been a girlie-girl or a womany-woman and, like marriage, motherhood had never really been on my to-do list either. How on earth would I cope with a baby when I was getting up at 3.30 every morning? And I'd only been in the job about eighteen months – would the top brass at *GMTV* think I wasn't committed to the role? Nothing could have been further from the truth. On top of that, what on earth did I know about babies? I preferred going out for dinner or watching football. Still, a baby was on its way so it was clearly meant to be – we just had to make it work somehow.

I couldn't face telling anyone at work as I was terrified I'd be out on my ear. In those days, pregnant women were virtually an invisible breed on television. When Anne Diamond first appeared on TV-am's *Good Morning Britain* with a baby bump just over ten years earlier, in 1987, half the viewers' heads nearly fell off! And maternity policy wasn't anything like it is now. There were no guarantees *GMTV* would hold my job open while I was away.

Tellingly, I was as concerned about breaking the news to Mum and Dad as I was about informing my bosses. I just felt sort of guilty. I knew Mum and Dad really needed me – that's why I was up and down the M4 at weekends like a yo-yo. Mum seemed so lost and alone. Would she think that by having a baby, I was abandoning her in favour of my new life?

By that Christmas, my bump was showing. Martin and I were nervous about the thought of becoming parents, but incredibly excited too. Yet still I couldn't bring myself to tell Mum I was pregnant. To me, it seemed she was so disinterested in my life nowadays, she didn't deserve to know.

Martin and I drove down to Wales to spend Christmas with Mum and Dad but, when we arrived, there was no food in the fridge and only a rather sickly looking, sparsely decorated tree stood in the corner. I still felt it was Mum and Dad's marital standoff that meant neither of them wanted to make an effort, despite their kids and partners having made the effort to be there. In the end, we went out to buy crisps and a bottle of wine, then sat around chatting while Mum withdrew quietly in the corner, like an outsider in her own family.

A couple of days later, Martin and I were still there after my brothers had gone home. We went out for lunch with Mum and Dad to a pub by the beach in a beautiful village called Dale. When Mum went to the toilet, Martin and I told Dad about the baby.

He was pleased.

'I don't think it's quite the right time to tell Mum, though,' I said hesitantly.

'Why?' asked Dad, appearing to be totally baffled that I thought there was a problem.

He didn't seem to think there was anything unusual about

her behaviour. Maybe he was so used to the way she was by then that he no longer noticed. Or perhaps he had just shut down the ability to see how changed she was.

I was angry that Mum was acting so cold towards me – did she resent me having a life with Martin in London and a career that made me happy? I just didn't know.

The four of us walked along the beach after our lunch and finally I put my arm through hers and broke the news: 'Mum, I'm having a baby.'

'Oh, that's lovely,' she said. 'When's it due?'

But that was about it. No wild excitement, no giggling over her favourite baby names, no conversation about how on earth I'd manage being a mum with work – she was just blank.

Mum was sixty-six then, which is still relatively young, but it was like she had already opted out of life. While most women that age would be thrilled at the prospect of becoming a granny, she seemed utterly unbothered. It was another trip to my parents that ended in me swinging between rage and tears on the way home. The longer I spent with them, the more their depression and emptiness spread to me – or so it felt. It was a relief to return to London, yet still something always pulled me back to them in Wales.

On 28 May 1999, my first son Nathaniel (Nat) was born at Chelsea and Westminster Hospital. I was still quite tiny, but Nat weighed in at a chunky 9lb 3oz.

All those years of thinking I'd never wanted a baby . . . but from the very first moment I saw my beautiful Nat, I was completely besotted. His tiny little fingernails, his soft baby smell, the way his eyes would open just a flicker and then close back to sleep again. He was perfect. Martin was enthralled too. We couldn't quite believe this was happening to us – a career-driven, independent couple. Suddenly, we were obsessed parents, spending every moment worrying about whether Nat was feeding enough, whether he needed burping or a nappy change, whether he was warm enough or too warm, whether his baby seat was properly secured. There were a million new things to worry about. How on earth were we – with absolutely no experience – being entrusted with this beautiful little thing? But there was also a vivid sense that we were now a family.

We were on cloud nine but, sure enough, Mum and Dad soon punctured that feeling. When I rang to tell them that the baby had arrived, Dad answered the phone.

'It's a boy!' I said.

'Oh, fantastic, that's great news,' he said. 'I'll get your mum.'

At which point I started gushing again: 'Hi, Mum, he's arrived . . . It's a boy!'

And then nothing. Silence on the line.

'A little boy,' I repeated.

I couldn't quite hear what she was saying, but then I heard her mumble: 'Ah well, maybe the next one will be a girl.'

I couldn't believe it. How could she be such an absolute cow? I'd just been through an excruciating labour, my hormones were racing faster than Evel Knievel, I was lying next to the most beautiful baby that had ever been born and my mum sounded disappointed? Even then, I didn't challenge her. I didn't call her

99

out for being so downright cruel. Instead, I just faked a laugh and said: 'You'll have to come and see him soon.'

But when I put the phone down, the tears came again. Why was she being so unkind?

A couple of weeks later, Mum did travel to London to see Nat. She was supposedly there to help me out as Martin had been sent as *GMTV* chief correspondent to report on the war in Kosovo. But quickly it felt like I had two babies to look after, not just one. First of all, Mum couldn't remember which was her bag when the coach pulled in at Victoria. Then, when we got back to our house, she struggled to make me a cup of tea while I fed Nat.

'You just flick that switch at the side of the kettle,' I snapped as Mum stood there looking at the kettle as if it was some strange bit of technology.

Everything was difficult and the worst of it was her general sense of disinterest.

'I wonder if she's jealous of Nat?' I said to Martin on the phone.

The thought that anyone could be jealous of my beautiful baby boy was infuriating. I probably wasn't the perfect daughter then either. Nat was a hungry baby and was waking several times a night to be breastfed. I felt shattered. But I couldn't even nap during the daytime as I felt I had to keep an eye on Mum.

One night after Martin had returned home and we were asleep in bed with Nat next to us in his Moses basket, the door opened and Mum walked in.

'Where am I?' she asked, looking utterly terrified.

'It's fine, Mum, you're with Martin and me,' I said, walking her back to her room.

Obviously, now, with hindsight, I can see how ill she must have been, but at the time I thought she was sleepwalking or so drugged up on Tamoxifen that it was messing with her mind.

I got Mum back to bed, went back to sleep myself and sure enough, fifteen minutes later, Nat was awake for his next feed. It was exhausting.

Another time, David and his wife and Andrew and his then-girlfriend came over to see the new baby. Everyone was drinking and chatting in the garden, but Mum went indoors to sit by herself in the kitchen, so I came to check on her.

'What's the matter, Mum?' I asked.

'No one's interested in me,' she said.

'Don't be daft,' I told her, 'everyone's always interested in you.'

I laughed, but inside I was raging. How dare she think she was in competition with a one-month-old baby? *My* one-month-old baby.

I was relieved when she went home. She'd done nothing to help. Friends of mine had mums who would look after their babies so they could get a break, go out for dinner or return to work. My mum barely looked at Nat, let alone gave me a break or offered to cook dinner.

Four months after giving birth to Nat, I was back sitting next to Eamonn Holmes on the *GMTV* sofa. The team was brilliant and welcomed me back, even humouring me by looking at all my baby photos. But I knew I couldn't have stayed away any longer – I was terrified that, if I had, they'd have forgotten I existed and drafted in some bright young thing instead. Leaving my gorgeous baby that first day at 4 a.m. in the pitch-dark was heart-wrenching. I had tears running down my face when I got in the cab to take me into the studio. A massive part of me just wanted to sit at home holding my baby for ever.

But you've always worked, you've got to work, I told myself.

Mentally, I had backed myself into a corner where I thought I had no option. For those first few months I would dash home at the end of my shift to feed Nat and spend every moment I could with him until his bath and bedtime. Then I'd be straight into bed myself in the desperate hope I'd get a couple of hours' uninterrupted sleep before something started screaming – either my alarm clock or my baby.

11

Mum visited frequently during the first year of Nat's life. Each time I hoped the trip would be more successful than the last – it rarely was.

During one of her stays, I realized that her GP must have put her on antidepressants when I saw a packet she had left in the bathroom.

'Well, if they make you feel better, it's worth a go,' I said, though I wasn't convinced – my dislike of tablets to fix problems might not be fashionable, but it is deep-rooted within me. I wanted Mum better, but it worried me that the Seroxat drug – one of a group of medicines called SSRIs (selective serotonin reuptake inhibitors) – she had been prescribed could have nasty side effects. Some believed it could even cause suicidal tendencies – how was that going to help a deeply unhappy and depressed woman?

On one of her visits I left Mum at a salon to get her hair done while I popped to the shops. When I returned to meet her, she'd already gone.

'We finished early so she just left,' the stylist said.

I felt a gut-sinking panic. Mum didn't know this area of London and she could be anywhere. Pushing Nat in the buggy, I ran up and down the street. The level of panic I felt must have indicated that deep down, I knew there was a serious problem. It wasn't a toddler who had just wandered off, this was a woman in her sixties.

Finally, I found Mum casually wandering along a side road.

'Oh, you're there, what a relief,' I said, trying to hide the utter panic in my voice. She just looked at me blankly, as if I was making a fuss about nothing. Or maybe because she just didn't know why I would be worried.

Nat had just turned one when I took him down to Wales for a weekend. It was then that things finally, finally started to fall into place. Mum had left her diary out open on the kitchen worktop. It was a total mess of scribblings, crossed-out appointments and 'Doctor' written in capital letters on lots and lots of dates.

'What's all these trips to the doctor about, Mum?' I asked.

'Oh, I'm not sure,' she replied hesitantly. 'I really can't remember.'

It might sound strange, but I believed her – I didn't think she was lying to me, but that she was confused or had been a bit muddled maybe by some technical diagnosis.

'OK, I'll come with you for the next appointment then,' I said.

A few days later, we walked into the surgery together and although it might sound incredible now, I had absolutely no idea what the GP was about to say.

'We think your mother might have Alzheimer's disease,' the doctor said.

Mum didn't say anything; she just kept staring mutely ahead.

'Oh, I don't think so,' I replied. 'She's only in her sixties and that's what old people get. And she's been depressed for a long time. Things aren't great between her and my dad and it's all got on top of her.'

'That may be the case,' the doctor said kindly, 'but our tests are pointing towards Alzheimer's.'

We left no further forward. I didn't think Mum could possibly have Alzheimer's. Even if she did, the doctor didn't seem to have any idea what to do about it. And Mum didn't seem to be thinking anything at all.

Back in London I took to googling everything I could possibly find about the disease. Yes, she fitted the bill on things like memory loss, but there were other times when her memory was OK so that didn't seem like her. The internet also revealed the absolute horror of Alzheimer's: it is terminal. If that's what she had, there was nothing that could be done to prevent its steady advance. I wouldn't – I couldn't – accept that was what was happening. And also, I told myself, many of her symptoms didn't tally with Alzheimer's.

The big issue was her being so withdrawn and depressed. Every time I rang her now, she would cry on the phone. I felt so guilty that I started travelling down to see her every weekend when I finished work. I'd strap little Nat into his car seat and head off down the M4. But when I got there, Mum quite often didn't even seem as though she could be bothered to talk to me. Dad would be sitting in his chair watching the telly, seemingly totally disengaged from what was going on.

Why on earth do I bother? I'd seethe to myself, trying to get their house straight in between feeding Nat and preparing for another busy week back on the *GMTV* sofa on Monday morning.

I decided that I would accompany Mum to an appointment with a hospital consultant about Alzheimer's. He told me she had taken two memory tests and the most recent one showed a sharp decline in her cognitive ability.

'But she's depressed,' I kept saying. 'My parents have an awful relationship and she can't cope.'

He shook his head. 'I'm afraid during the tests we ask questions like the name of the prime minister or which month it is and she didn't know.'

'But that's because she's depressed,' I insisted.

'We really don't believe that is all,' he said. 'We firmly believe this is Alzheimer's.'

I kept thinking about what I'd read online – if this was Alzheimer's it meant my mum wasn't coming back. Ever. Mum was still only sixty-six years old. It was all so incredibly, monstrously unfair. And all that time I'd thought she had depression and this was just a phase that she and Dad would get through and she'd return to be my funny, bubbly, smiling mum. But now this consultant at the desk was telling me that woman was gone for ever.

My mum had left me. She was never, ever coming back.

Meanwhile, what he was saying to Mum didn't register at all – she just continued to sit there for the fifteen-minute appointment, looking at her watch.

Afterwards, I got her in the car and drove us home, blinking as hard as I could to stop the tears pouring down my face. In the months ahead, there were so many tears as we came to terms with her diagnosis and she lost more of her grip on life. There was the time she started crying in the supermarket because she couldn't remember why she was there or where they stocked the bread. Then when we were walking down the street together and we bumped into her friend. Despite chatting away about the weather and how the children were, after she walked off, Mum turned to me with tears in her eyes – she had no idea who they were. And there was the time she rang me at home in London in the middle of the night, sobbing: 'Please help me. Please.'

She was so terrified and it was agonizing to hear that terror constantly in her voice.

Dad just seemed to be standing back from everything that was going on – it was almost as if it had nothing to do with him. He was still working and out of the house for hours every day, much as he had been throughout our childhood. During the day Mum stayed indoors alone, increasingly too scared of the outside world to venture out.

The GP put her on Aricept, a drug that was meant to slow the advance of Alzheimer's. I think it did a bit – and some days she could put a brave face on what she was going through – but the medication gave her stomach cramps and did nothing to help with her depression.

Things limped on. Mum became gradually worse, forgetting how to cook and clean, and Dad grew more impatient and frustrated.

'That bloody woman,' he'd seethe when she sat in her chair, silently weeping.

'Dad, she's not well. It's Alzheimer's, it's a disease,' I'd try to tell him. But he didn't listen, he'd just chunter on to himself.

Sometimes his anger towards Mum would bubble to the surface and he would yell at her and she'd just cry more. Because us kids were all living away from home and Dad wasn't coping with the situation, leaving Mum to fend for herself, the local GP helped make contact with social workers. They sent Dad on an anger-management course, but the atmosphere in the house remained fraught. Trips down to Wales were emotionally exhausting, but when I heard my mum crying down the phone I felt I had to go.

There was another eight years between Mum's diagnosis and when she passed away from Alzheimer's. We will never know for certain how long she had it before the official diagnosis or how long she had felt something changing within herself and had hidden it from the rest of the family. My feeling, though, is that it may have stretched back to when she was fifty-three or fifty-four, which was so, so young.

Perhaps it was the sense of guilt that I hadn't picked up sooner on what was happening to Mum that made me so determined to care for her as best I could after she was diagnosed. I also felt bad for being so far away in London. Ultimately, I was determined to care for her and spend as much time as I could with her because she was my lovely, lovely mum and I loved her. There was nothing she wouldn't have done for us when we were kids. She had sacrificed everything for her family yet her husband was emotionally distant and her three children were off living their own lives. I felt wracked with sorrow and guilt about my poor mum being so isolated, alone and scared of the illness over-whelming her. So began the trips back and forth to Wales almost every weekend.

I became so rundown myself from the early mornings at work, combined with caring for Nat and visiting Mum, that I came down with shingles and had to have three weeks off work. I could barely get out of bed. My weight plummeted until I was wearing size-six clothes and I lost all energy.

The cruel impact of Alzheimer's was hitting our entire family.

Then Mum was offered a week away in a respite care home. I think the social workers must have decided my parents needed some time apart as their relationship was so awful. Dad and I drove Mum to the home in Milford Haven. It was a pretty place with a view out over the water, but she was terrified by it all.

'You just want to get rid of me,' she said, physically trembling.

'Of course I don't, Mum,' I told her. 'We just thought this could be a nice place for a proper rest while they sort you out.'

Walking away as she cried and begged us to take her with us was horrendous. Even Dad looked upset that time. I felt sick with guilt and sadness and anger at the whole situation.

In the autumn of 2001, I found out that I was pregnant again. It was a bit of good news amid the worry. Martin and I were delighted there'd be a new brother or sister for Nat. At the same time, I had absolutely no idea how we'd manage with two little kids and our full-on jobs: one baby had been tough enough, but two?

By then, Martin had been promoted to editor of *GMTV*, which was an incredible opportunity, but we both felt the need to be more diligent than ever. We didn't want people to ever think we were taking advantage of our marriage to get away with not doing our absolute best. And it could be a bit awkward, being married to the boss! I don't think Eamonn Holmes loved the idea of my husband becoming editor. He never said anything explicitly and seemed to really like Martin, but after he was promoted, my relationship with Eamonn was never quite the same again.

Mum, Dad, my two brothers and their families came to visit for Christmas that year. On Boxing Day, Dad took his dog Bizzy for a walk. Two hours later, he still hadn't returned and that was when I started to worry. Finally, the doorbell rang. Dad was standing there with a police officer. Bizzy had been off the lead and was somehow hit by a car. He was OK though shaken, but Dad was in a real state.

'I was worried about your dad,' the policeman said. 'He seemed disorientated and couldn't remember where he was going. All he could say was your name.'

Honestly, this was the last thing I needed. I was pregnant, the house was full of people, including a toddler and an ill mother, and now my dad was wandering off. Fortunately, the policeman knew I lived in the area and had brought him home. 'Thank you so, so much,' I kept saying to the officer who had really gone out of his way to help.

The following day, Dad seemed more back to normal, or at least his grumpy, angry normal. Once again, there was an enormous great warning flag being waved, but I didn't see it.

I was just weeks away from giving birth when I got a phone call at work from the police saying there had been an 'incident' at Mum and Dad's house. Dad had snapped again and totally lost his temper with Mum. It was so bad that a neighbour had called the police to calm things down.

Livid, I rang home and Mum answered, crying once again.

'Get him on the phone!' I demanded.

Dad came on.

'What the bloody hell have you been doing?' I yelled. 'She's fucking ill, don't you realize?'

I'd never sworn like that at my dad before, but I was at breaking point by then.

'I'm ill too!' he yelled back.

'Don't be ridiculous!' I snapped. That was typical of Dad, always playing the victim. Or so I thought at the time.

I didn't know it then but the first signs that Dad was also suffering from Alzheimer's had begun. He was only sixty-six, again so young. Maybe it was because he was still young and active that I didn't see his behaviour for what it was. And surely lightning couldn't strike twice in such a terrible, terrible way?

On 14 May 2002, our second son – Mackenzie – was born just half an hour after a dash in the middle of the night to the Chelsea and Westminster Hospital. I was so, so fortunate. Again I had a perfect, beautiful baby in my arms. Things could still be good too. But this time there was no way Mum would be coming to visit to 'help' with the newborn – her condition had gone further downhill.

Mackenzie was only six weeks old when I got a call to say that Mum had fallen over at home, broken her hip and was being looked after in hospital. For the umpteenth time, that weekend Martin and I drove down the M4 – this time with two babies buckled up in the back of the car.

I was holding Mackenzie when I walked onto the hospital ward, hoping a glimpse of her newest grandson might give Mum a bit of a lift. But what I saw when I walked in was one of the most shocking moments of that whole time. Mum was lying in bed, but her body kept jerking violently from one position to another. She wasn't focusing on anything and was in some kind of stupor – the broken hip was the least of her problems.

For the very first time I understood Mum wasn't going to be getting better. In fact, she was dying. For years I'd kidded myself about her condition because I didn't want to believe it, but I couldn't deny it any longer. And then Mackenzie started screaming for a feed. It was all just too much.

Mum's hip gradually recovered, but she didn't. I don't know if it was the effects of the general anaesthetic for the op or a sudden deterioration in her condition, but she lost the ability to speak properly and instead just made sounds with the occasional word. She cried and cried. Dad said he couldn't cope with having her back home so we started to look at residential care. Martin and I talked about whether she could come and live with us if we got carers in to help, but with both of us working full-time and two little babies it just didn't seem doable.

Finally, David and I visited a home called Fairfield, a mile from where Mum and Dad lived. It seemed great. But I was consumed with guilt that we were abandoning Mum to be cared for by strangers. I tried to deal with that by driving down with the boys almost every weekend, not that she ever really understood we were there. She had gone past the point of being able to recognize us when we walked in.

I was utterly exhausted all the time. The 3.30 a.m. starts, the weekend drives, the constant tiredness. I had also taken on a role as an ambassador for the Alzheimer's Society – appearing at events, fronting advertising campaigns and speaking publicly on the issue. It took up quite a bit of time and emotional energy, but I felt it was something I could do in memory of Mum. On top of all that, Mackenzie developed severe eczema, which would wake him throughout the night as he tried to scratch at his inflamed skin.

It was all too much; I was a wreck.

I didn't confide in anyone at work because I just wanted

them to see the workaholic professional, getting on with the job. But maybe I wasn't doing as good a job at that as I thought. Eamonn Holmes and I would always have a chat and a cup of tea after the show and one day he turned to me and said, 'You're severely depressed, you've got too much to cope with.'

'I'm fine,' I laughed, always my response to everything.

With all that was going on I didn't have time to be depressed. I had to keep going for everyone's sake. If I did think about what was going on it was only to ask myself, *Why can't you manage all this? You just need to work a bit harder.*

Thinking about it now, I must have been totally mad but, amid all that, in 2005, I agreed to take part in the BBC's *Strictly Come Dancing*. My agent had been approached to see if I would be interested in appearing in the show's first series in the summer of 2004, but no one had any idea what the programme would be like back then and prancing around on prime-time TV didn't seem like my kind of thing. Then they came back and asked me to join the second series in the autumn of that year. By then the whole country had fallen in love with the show. I was a massive fan too but, having watched how much rehearsal time went into preparing for the live performances each week, I really didn't think it was for me. Again, I said no.

But my agent had other thoughts. When the request came in again for the third series, she was adamant: 'If you don't do it now, you can say goodbye to big gigs at the BBC – and you might need them one day if things go wrong at *GMTV*. Also, you need your bosses now to know you're in demand elsewhere.

It's the only way they'll appreciate you. I really think you ought to do it.'

And so I reluctantly agreed and signed up for the third series of *Strictly* in the autumn of 2005. Even as a teenager I had hated getting on the dance floor, so the whole thing was terrifying, but I gritted my teeth and tried to make the most of it. There were moments of the show that I really loved, but a lot of it was gruelling. I was still doing the early starts and trying to see Mum while looking after two kids under six. And now I had hours of dance practice to squeeze in every day too.

On the first week I was paired with the professional dancer, Brendan Cole. I think he soon found me a huge disappointment. He was a very hard taskmaster and determined to win. I was massively out of my comfort zone and, to be honest, not very good. I think it must have driven him mad. A story even appeared in the newspapers claiming Brendan had called me 'the worst partner he'd ever had'.

Charming!

In reality, though, it was probably true – but then wasn't the whole idea supposed to be about people who can't dance learning how to do it? OK, I admit I was pretty bad. I quickly became one of the series' comedy characters, like Ann Widdecombe or John Sergeant. And while I could laugh that off when we were on camera, I don't think deep down anyone really wants to be consistently the joke contestant.

A couple of years ago, when there was all the talk about bullying behind the scenes at *Strictly*, some rehearsal footage emerged where Brendan was seen shouting and swearing at the film crew. He could also be seen looking at my dancing, saying, 'Pathetic, it's not good enough!' Then I'm begging him to 'stop shouting' and worrying that I look completely ridiculous. There's a clip where I say to the cameraman that Brendan is looking at me like he's stepped in something.

I really don't remember much of that time now – maybe I blocked it out because all I recall is the sense that it was incredibly traumatic. I was on the brink of tears most of the time and felt utterly exhausted. And it all seemed so pointless. Brendan would be swinging me around the dance floor for a paso doble (or whatever the hell they call it) and I'd be thinking, *I've just put Mum in a care home, what on earth am I doing dressed up to the nines in a dancing competition?*

I should probably have told the crew – or even Brendan – how much I was struggling, but I didn't. I just stumbled on. Literally. And I didn't have time to seek help elsewhere, even if I'd been able to admit that I needed it.

Fortunately (although I don't think Brendan saw it that way), we were voted out in Week Four. It was all over on Bonfire Night. What a relief! Soon afterwards, Mum was readmitted to hospital – she had become very weak. I hurtled back down the M4 to find her alone and unconscious in the hospital bed. She didn't even have a nightie with her.

When I got to the hospital, I rang Dad, who'd barely visited Mum since she moved into the care home. The only time he would go was if I picked him up, took him there, then dropped him home again afterwards. After forty-five years of marriage he seemed to have totally abdicated all responsibility for his wife. That was why I felt so much responsibility. My brothers were living at the other end of the country and would make trips to Wales whenever they could, but they had full-time jobs and their own lives to lead too.

'Are you coming to visit Mum?' I asked Dad.

'I can't – I'm busy fixing my bike,' he said.

'I'll come and fetch you then?'

'No, it's OK, thanks.'

There must have been a million times when I thought I'd had it with Dad, but that really was the final straw. How could he be so cruel?

Unable to walk or talk properly, Mum went back to the care home soon after. Her world had shrunk smaller and smaller, bounded only by fear and pain. Then just before midnight on 14 May 2006, the phone rang at home. It had been Mackenzie's fourth birthday and I was in bed because there would be another early start on *GMTV*.

It was the care home to say Mum was seriously ill and maybe I should travel down to say goodbye. I'd had a similar call several times before and yet she kept clinging on.

I tossed and turned all night, not certain what was the right thing to do. Then, when the alarm went off at four, I decided I had to go. What if she did die in the care home without any family around her while I was smiling and chatting away to strangers on the television?

I struggle to remember much of this now, maybe because it was so upsetting, but I recently reread what I wrote shortly afterwards:

When I arrived, she was in her room, just lying there. And I knew it was the end. I kissed her and knew I was never going to take her on our much-discussed coach trip to Holland to see the tulip fields, that we'd never ever talk and talk and talk, never laugh till we fell over. I sat on her small single bed, with the rubber sheets and cheap pillows, and I wanted to scream for all her pain and the tears, for the not being able to help, for the guilt at handing her over to someone else's care when she'd loved and cared for me so much. For the guilt I knew would never leave me, for all the horrible things I'd ever said or done, for not letting her know every day that I loved her. I held her hand and cradled what was left of her.

All day I sat there by the bed, then I stayed in the hotel and returned again the following morning until the late afternoon and still she clung on. I couldn't decide whether to stay or go. I spoke to my brother David, who was also a regular visitor to Mum, and he said, 'Go home to your boys.' One of the lovely nurses at the care home who I'd got to know came and sat with me.

'Your mum went years ago,' she said, 'we'll look after her now.'

And so, in the end, I got back in the car and drove back to London.

I'd barely got in the door when the care home rang to say Mum had gone. She had died without me there to hold her. And of all the things I regret in my life, the greatest is that I wasn't with her at the end.

I hate Alzheimer's for that, for wearing you down and taking the person you love away from you bit by bit by bit so when it's the very final goodbye, you're too worn down to be there.

That evening, I rang Dad and then my brothers to pass on the news. Despite the terrible way he'd behaved for years and years, Dad seemed entirely crushed.

'I'll go up to the home to be with her,' he said quietly.

If only he'd done that over the past few years.

Mum's funeral was beautiful. Colleagues from the department store where she worked came along and all the friends she had chatted to before she became ill. For me there was just a sense of agonizing loss. Mum, my greatest champion, my constant support through everything, was gone – and I hadn't been able to stop it happening.

12

The guilt at not being able to do more to care for Mum had almost driven me mad. And there was still Dad – he needed looking after too.

He'd changed so much from the man I'd adored as a kid. He remained bitter at the way his life had turned out and as a result had withdrawn from it all. He was on antidepressants to help him sleep and moderate his moods, but they didn't seem to be doing much good.

I focused all my efforts on trying to care for Dad in a way I felt I had failed with Mum. My brothers thought I was punishing myself in trying to rebuild the shattered relationship between me and Dad. The boys accepted Dad at face value and thought he was just being difficult, as he had been so much during our childhood. They didn't seem to crave his approval in the way I still did. Maybe that's what comes of being the eldest child.

'You have to accept that he's never going to be who you want him to be,' David would say.

And although I knew rationally he was right, emotionally I couldn't quite do it.

A couple of months after Mum's death I went back down to Wales to spend some time with Dad. I didn't really feel he wanted me there – it was as if I was somehow intruding on his grief. When we talked over a coffee in a local cafe, he was tearful. He spoke as if the years Mum had been living in the care home had never happened and he had been a doting husband right to the end – it couldn't have been further from the truth. It seemed so utterly self-indulgent and overemotional to me, considering how he had behaved, but I didn't have the heart to tell him what I really thought.

Still then I was hoping he could be a better person.

When I went down, I stayed in a hotel as I got the feeling he didn't want the hassle of having to get a guest room ready. I rarely went to the house as he preferred to meet in a local cafe and I knew he didn't really enjoy cooking after Mum had stopped making dinner for them both.

Soon after Mum died, David and I took Dad to a solicitor to make a will and sort out some paperwork. Mum hadn't done any of that and it had made a difficult situation even worse when she became ill. We thought it was important for everyone to get on top of all that legal admin while we could.

Dad sat with the solicitor while David and I waited outside, but about ten minutes later we were called back in without him.

'I'm afraid your dad can't make a will,' the solicitor said. 'He can't remember all your names or even his own address, which means he's not sufficiently mentally fit to go ahead with it.'

'He's recently lost his wife and is very depressed,' I replied.

Looking back, I can see I was like a stuck record. I was

making exactly the same excuses for Dad's behaviour as I had for Mum, but there was no way at that time that I could see the same thing coming for us once again.

Not again.

But it was.

Over the next few months Dad would ring me in a panic about all sorts of things and I took over handling his bills and car insurance. Then a letter arrived one day from Dad. Instead of his usual confident handwriting it was a mix of lower- and upper-case characters and at the top of the envelope he'd written the words 'Fiona and Martin's address'. It was a warning sign, but still I thought maybe he was just depressed and had been knocked a bit off course by Mum's death. Nothing more.

A couple of months later I got a call from his GP saying they were a bit worried about Dad. He'd been back and forward to the pharmacy to collect a prescription, totally forgetting that he'd already collected it.

'We're worried he has some cognitive difficulties,' the doctor said.

'Yes, but he's depressed,' I replied once more although it was starting to fall into place – his strange behaviour during Mum's final illness, the way he wouldn't let us into the house, that time he'd got lost while staying with us in London and then recently not even being able to remember his own address at the solicitor's office.

'Oh no,' I said. 'You don't think it could be Alzheimer's, do you?'

'It could be,' the doctor replied. 'We'll need to do some tests.'

The tests proved everything we feared. Here we were again. And once again, the guilt was back – this time I felt guilty that I'd been so wrapped up in Mum's illness that I hadn't noticed Dad was becoming seriously ill too.

Dad was sixty-eight at this time and was to live for another six years after Mum. Another six years of worry and watching as a parent was stolen away from me. And once again I fell into the role of trying to make everything 'right'. Of course I couldn't – you can't make Alzheimer's 'right' – but I was carrying all that crushing responsibility of being the eldest child, and the only daughter, and the child who had so, so wanted us to be a happy family however elusive that could be.

Again, I was back to the weekly or fortnightly trips to Wales, fuelled by guilt to do whatever I could. Still, Dad didn't want me going in the house so instead, I'd stay in a hotel nearby and we'd go for walks or out for a pub lunch. I can't say he was ever delighted to see me but, once we were out, his mood would lift and he'd laugh and joke with the waiting staff. There was no doubt his memory was slipping, but he actually seemed lighter and less grumpy than he had been in years.

The illness was descending fast. The only positive to be taken from this repeating nightmare was that rather than seem sad and terrified as Mum had done, Dad appeared more jolly and good-humoured.

Alzheimer's had come for him, but in a very different way.

13

By the start of 2007, I'd been getting up for work each day at 3.30 a.m. for a decade. Nat was still just eight, Mackenzie was five. For the entire time I had been combining my role as a TV presenter with caring for my parents as best I could.

I was running on empty.

In 2005, Eamonn Holmes left *GMTV*, claiming the show had become 'celebrity-obsessed'. Eamonn was a good journalist, but not always the easiest person to work with. After he left, I became the show's 'veteran' host. It felt like a new opportunity for me. For years, if there was a big interview to be done with a politician, Eamonn would lead the conversation and I was supposed to chip in with a few questions near the end – I hated that.

I also discovered Eamonn had been paid significantly more than me. It seems incredible that well into this century, no one had batted an eyelid at a man being paid more than a woman for doing exactly the same job.

After Eamonn had left, Andrew Castle and then Ben Shephard joined me on the sofa. They were lovely to work with and I felt a bit more in control of how things went on the show, but the 3.30 a.m. starts never got any easier – in fact, they became a whole lot worse.

By then I was working three days a week on the show and packed my other days with work too. One of my favourite new jobs was the newspaper column I wrote, which appeared in the *Daily Mirror* every Saturday. When Piers Morgan was editor of the *Mirror*, he had invited me to lunch and we had a fairly frank exchange of views on all sorts of issues. Afterwards he sent me a very cheeky message and I sent one straight back, which put him in his place. His next message appeared a second later: 'Great reply – would you like a column in the *Mirror*?'

'OK, it's a deal,' I replied.

A couple of weeks later, my first full-page column appeared. I was so proud. Finally, I felt I was being regarded as a proper journalist. I was able to write about issues that really mattered to me, such as funding for health and the state of our education system, but I was able to keep readers entertained with showbiz gossip that I came across too.

I couldn't believe the response from readers. Each week I'd be flooded with lovely letters from people who had enjoyed the column. There were soon so many that we started a regular section called 'Ask Fiona', where readers could ask for my thoughts on anything at all. I loved it!

On top of the newspaper column, I was also presenting on BBC Radio London, on a new venture called *OK!TV* and on various one-off documentaries that came my way. Whenever work was offered, I felt a huge pressure to say 'Yes'.

I was very aware of how TV bosses think – I needed them to know other shows were interested in me so they wouldn't think I was a washed-up old has-been. So I piled more and more pressure – and work – on myself. Then I'd be dashing home from wherever I was working to pick the boys up from school, give them some tea and help them with their home-work before falling into bed and doing it all over again the next day.

The house felt like it was in a constant state, with football boots and school uniform scattered around. I hated that and was a bit obsessive about tidying up. And every time I passed a shop I had to load up on food because the family ate so much. I felt like I was rushing around doing everything, but not really succeeding at anything.

Martin and I rarely went out as a couple and when friends asked us around for dinner, my knee-jerk response was always, 'Oh God, what excuse can I give not to go?' because I was so tired. It was tiredness verging on an illness or at least that's how it felt anyway. Whatever it was, it wasn't normal. Even at home I never just sat down and relaxed or watched TV because I was trying to fit everything in. Maybe I'd become a bit manic. I could be dead on my feet with exhaustion but still fretting that I needed to knock up a moussaka because there were two aubergines in the fridge that needed using up.

I know people might say now, 'Why on earth didn't you turn down the extra work?' or 'Why didn't you get a cleaner and a housekeeper?', but I was stuck on a hamster wheel and I didn't know how to jump off.

Martin and I had the most horrendous rows. They'd blow up over something ridiculous like the state of the kitchen and why couldn't he empty the dishwasher or whatever, then spiral up from there.

'I need more help around the place, Martin!' I'd yell. 'You expect me to do everything.'

And then he'd come back at me: 'Well, what do you want me to do? Give up my job?'

'No, I just feel like it all comes down to me.'

'Well, let's get a live-in nanny then!' he'd yell, knowing full well my views on that.

'I don't want a live-in nanny taking over my house!' I'd shout back.

And then it would fade away for a bit. But once I saw we'd made Mackenzie cry because we were screaming at each other so much, I knew this wasn't healthy. The fact we were so frazzled all the time shouldn't have been making our children unhappy. I know this happens in families all the time when you're both working and kids are little, but for me it was just one more thing to feel guilty about.

And men just want simple solutions to problems, don't they? You're knackered – so give up work. You're constantly rushing to fetch the kids – then hire a nanny. You look a state – book a spa weekend. But life's not that simple. I was caught up in so many conflicting emotions: I knew the job was destroying me, but it gave me security and purpose too. I knew I wasn't giving the boys the attention they needed, but I didn't want to pay someone else to do that when I'd been brought up to believe that was my job alone. And I loved Martin and our family, so why couldn't I just stop yelling at everyone?

By then I'd lost control of my own life and was just clinging to whatever direction it took me in like a child clinging to a sledge as it hurtles down a hill with no idea where it's going to end up. I think I was probably depressed too although unable to recognize it myself – I could cry at the merest things and often I'd be crying when we had guests telling emotional stories at work. Then I'd go back to my dressing room and cry some more because I just felt so disconnected to my life.

I was exhausted and pictures of me walking down the street looking shattered never failed to please the women's magazines. Around then I was constantly on their front covers with head-lines saying something ridiculous like 'New heartache for Fiona'. There was no heartache, I was just knackered, but appar-ently it did well for sales – it certainly didn't do much for my self-esteem. And so, in the summer of 2008, when I got wind that senior management wanted to shake up the show – and I wasn't part of their plans for what shook back down – I'd lost my energy to fight it.

That summer, we had another incredible three-week holiday on the Isle of Mull. We both loved the place. The children could spend hours playing in rock pools and we would go for long walks no matter the weather – it made it easier to think. That holiday, I did a lot of thinking about what I really wanted while there was a bit of calm in my life.

I knew it was time to walk away, but the thought of not being at *GMTV* was also terrifying. Leaving meant waving goodbye to job security and the familiarity of the place and all the people. I'd been so closely associated with that one show, would anyone else want me? I could be stepping into oblivion. But on that holiday, I was so carefree. I had energy for messing around with the kids and I knew if I could have that all the time it would mean so much to them – and my dad. Not to mention Martin. If I wasn't so permanently exhausted, maybe I could be a bit nicer to him.

On the Isle of Mull, I felt freer than I had in years. The thought of returning to that squeezed-in, squashed-in, hunched feeling where everything was dominated by the clock made me feel sick. My thoughts were incredibly conflicted and while I didn't want it any longer, I was still heartbroken to leave *GMTV* – I loved that job. But I'd been around long enough to know that in TV nothing stays the same for long and I'd had a very good run. Also, I really did feel that I needed to be around a bit more for the boys – and when I was there not to be constantly smiling through a fog of exhaustion.

Back in London, I agreed a deal with the bosses that meant I would leave at the end of the year. My last show was to be aired on 18 December 2008 – almost twelve years since my first day on that famous sofa.

There was a terrible trend then of stories about presenters being leaked to the press so it was decided that a statement would be released quickly and put out before the rumours spread. In the statement, I tried to be honest with the viewers who'd watched me all those years. I wrote: 'I love the job, but I've got other responsibilities – the children, a home life and an elderly dad who needs me – and I've recognized that I can't have it all.' But in the rush of it all I didn't really think those words through properly. What I should have said was: 'You can't have it all on 3.30 a.m. starts.'

Which is what I was feeling.

Either way, it led to a massive hoo-ha in the press. I came under attack from some people who said I'd let down other working women, but that was the last thing I wanted to do. What I wanted to scream was: 'You try getting up at 3.30 a.m. every morning for twelve years; 6.30 a.m. would be a breeze, 3.30 a.m. is hell – suck it and see!' The worst thing you could accuse me of is being a shirker – I push myself, I punish myself. I had reached a point where I felt a responsibility to my children – to be there for them, to take them to school, bring them home and not be constantly shattered and irritable. But then other people in the press used me as a stick to beat working women with, as if I was saying mothers should just be sitting at home or baking cakes.

This couldn't have been further from what I believed.

It was such a shame because what I really felt was far more nuanced than the press wanted to hear. Maybe women can have it all, but that means they have to *do* it all and then they haven't got it all anyway because they're so exhausted, they're not living life properly. That's my true take on it – 'having it all' is a compromise, it really is.

Apart from accidentally standing on the landmine of what society thinks about working women, the remainder of the response to my plan to leave was incredible. There were the most wonderful messages from people I'd interviewed over the years. I received a beautiful bouquet and card from Helen Newlove, the widow of Garry who was kicked to death by three drunk youths outside his home in 2007. I'd interviewed Helen many years ago about the incredible work she had gone on to do to represent victims of crime. And I had a lovely letter from Madeleine McCann's grandfather, offering support and thanking me for the way we had covered the awful case of that poor little girl's disappearance. I had interviewed Madeleine's parents, Gerry and Kate, on the show in 2008 when they were going through the most dreadful time. Even Tony Blair wrote me a letter saying: 'You were and are a superb professional, but also one of the nicest people I met in my time in UK politics.'

Each message I read had me collapsing into tears all over again. And then there were hundreds and hundreds of lovely letters from viewers who I suppose had just got used to waking up with me over the past twelve years. After the show I'd sit in my dressing room and cry as I read all the kind things people said about me.

I thought the boys would be delighted that I'd be around a bit more. Maybe they secretly were, but when I first told Mackenzie he couldn't believe it.

'You've quit TV?' he said, outraged. 'Who does that? Frank Lampard would never do that!'

And obviously at that time, in our Chelsea-obsessed home, what Frank would or wouldn't do was the guide to life! I explained that I wanted to spend more time with him and Nat, but that just led to a whole lot of eye-rolling. Sometimes I wonder if for working mums it's not actually the kids who miss out as much as we mothers do. Maybe the guilt we carry is more to do with what society has told us we ought to be doing, rather than what the kids themselves actually want or need.

In the run-up to the final show, I did another round of media interviews looking back at my time on *GMTV*. As I write this book, I am reading them all again to try to remember how I was feeling at that time. Clearly struggling, I was quite open about that with anyone who asked. I told one interviewer: 'I just can't wait to come up into daylight and see what's on the surface – it will be such a crushing blow if I'm still the same after I leave all this.'

Lovely Ben Shephard was co-presenting with me that final day and never left my side on the sofa as he knew how hard I was finding it and how close I was to dissolving into tears at any moment. There were recorded messages from Gordon Brown, David Cameron and Nick Clegg, Frank Lampard, Kate Winslet and Bruce Forsyth. I'd interviewed them all over the years and their messages were so kind – it was a bit like watching my own funeral!

All the formative things in my life had happened while I'd been on *GMTV* – I'd met and married Martin, I'd had my two boys, my mum had died and my dad had fallen ill. When I look back at the clip of my last day on the show, I say all that to the viewers at home. But in that list the first thing I mention is Mum dying – as if that had become the biggest issue in my life at that time, overwhelming so much else. Right at the end I told the viewers: 'It has been such a privilege sharing my mornings with you, but I need to be with my children and my dad and my husband – and be nice to him, for once! I will never forget your kindness.'

And then that was it. I stepped out of the studio for the last time. There was a lovely lunch afterwards with the rest of the team and then I went home to wrap the boys' Christmas presents. I was heartbroken and cried my way through the next few days, but there was also a quiet sense of calm. I was no longer public property to be peered at in magazines or judged for my every move – that was a relief.

14

I began the New Year of 2009, ready for a great new adventure. I threw myself into being the mum I'd never really had time to be before. I took the boys to school every morning and even had time for a chat with the other mothers on the school run. That had been impossible in the past and I loved it.

Meanwhile, I was being offered every kind of reality show you can think of – *I'm a Celebrity . . . Get Me Out of Here!*, *MasterChef* and *Celebrity Big Brother*, among many others – but my experience with *Strictly* had been quite enough. That sort of thing really didn't interest me. Without wishing to sound pompous, I wanted to make television that mattered. I started work on lots of documentary ideas, including one for Channel 4 and a film for *Panorama* called *Finished at Fifty?* I was determined that I definitely wasn't going to be finished after fifty! And I did get one very interesting offer of a new career opportunity in late 2007, which I certainly wasn't expecting. We were all at home one morning when Martin's phone rang.

'Good morning, I'm calling from number 10 Downing Street,' said the voice on the other end. 'I do hope you don't mind us ringing you, Martin, but we don't have Fiona's number and the Prime Minister would like to speak to her.'

The Prime Minister?

Martin called me to the phone, whispering in that wildly theatrical way that people do, 'It's Gordon Brown. On the phone. He wants to talk to *you*.'

Me?

And it was. I'd met Gordon quite a few times when he had been on *This Morning* and I had hugely admired him. He was – and is – a man of enormous integrity. We'd also met a few years earlier when Tony Blair was still prime minister and Martin and I were invited to the country home, Chequers, for dinner. That was such a funny night. Martin and I were giggling like school kids when we drove up the long track to the PM's official residence in the Buckinghamshire countryside.

It all sounded so grand – it was the kind of event Mum would have been beside herself to hear I had been invited to attend. But inside it was very underwhelming. The place looked slightly shabby and all decked out in the kind of decor you'd find around your granny's house. Whoever is prime minister also has to pay for any food and drink that is served there too. So there we were surrounded by historic oil paintings of the Duke of This and the Earl of That, and we were drinking £4.99 bottles of plonk from Tesco! Not that Martin and I cared – we had a great old time.

And that was the first time I'd met Gordon. We shared a lot of similar beliefs about how a good society should care for those who most need it and we talked a lot about education. I told him about how bad my comprehensive school had been but how I was entirely opposed to private education, which creates such a division within our society. I was adamant both our boys would have a state education like their parents. But that had been a good few years earlier so I was still bewildered as to why Gordon Brown, who'd become prime minister in 2007, was ringing me.

He quickly explained that he wanted to offer me a place within his government as an adviser on health issues. He said he had seen all the work I had done on the issue of Alzheimer's and asked if I would be interested in going in to number 10 to discuss the idea further.

'Yes, of course,' I replied, not really knowing what I'd be letting myself in for.

A series of meetings followed and Gordon was always lovely, utterly charming. It was at the time when he was trying to construct what was being called 'a government of all the talents' – a mixture of people with real world experience, not just politicians. If I'd taken the role, the plan was for me to be put forward for a peerage to join the House of Lords. It all sounded terribly exciting and I was incredibly flattered to be asked by someone who felt I could make a difference to the country, but I also knew it would mean a return to working long hours – and particularly late nights as so much of the voting and debates in Parliament go on well into the evening. And I wasn't ready to totally give up television work then either, which is what I'd have had to do because at that time there was no way you could be involved in politics and be on TV – it was deemed too much of a conflict of interest.

For weeks I mulled it over, but in the end I decided that having just found a bit of space in my life, it wasn't the right time for me to take on what would be an all-consuming job. I still loved all the chats I had with Gordon and I treasured that time I had getting to know him. Another deciding factor was I was trying to spend as much time as possible with Dad as his condition was worsening.

On my regular trips to Wales I would often meet Dad at a local hotel for lunch and I'd stay the night there while he went home. As I've said earlier, I got the strong sense he didn't want me in the house. It was a bit hurtful, but he'd always valued his independence and I thought that was the issue. If ever I popped around to the house to collect him for a trip out, he'd either not be there or would be waiting on the doorstep – there was never an invite in for a cup of tea and a biscuit.

As the months passed, I became a bit more suspicious about his behaviour – just what was he trying to hide? One day when I was dropping him back to the house, I made a point of saying I was coming in.

'Oh, you don't need to see me in the door,' Dad said.

'But I want to – I just want to check you get in and get the lights on OK,' I replied, quite firmly.

At that point a sense of resignation seemed to wash over him. It was like a child who is almost happy that they've been found out doing something they shouldn't be doing because the lying is over.

Dad opened the front door and I followed him down the hallway. What I saw when we got into the front room was horrendous. There was a filthy mattress on the living-room floor, which was where he must have been sleeping. All around it were piled clothes and papers. In the kitchen there were dirty pots and pans and plates that hadn't been washed up and half-eaten tins of food. It was awful. As I walked around the house taking it all in, I found notes written in his handwriting – some of it in capitals, some in lowercase, littered with the kind of spelling mistakes Dad would never have made before. They said things like 'Switch off kettle' and 'Turn off tap' (next to the sink). He was having to write these messages to remind himself to do simple everyday tasks; he must have known his memory loss was accelerating fast.

'Oh, Dad,' I said, 'why didn't you tell me you were struggling to cope?'

He looked so vulnerable and lost, but there was a definite sense of relief in his eyes: he didn't have to pretend any longer.

'Don't worry,' I told him. 'I'll get you out of here.'

'Thank you, Fiona,' he said. 'Thank you.'

My strong-willed, independent, tough Dad now looked so overwhelmed and childlike.

It took a few months longer than I'd hoped, but with help from Dad's brother, my Uncle Barry, we found him a lovely little flat in a warden-controlled home near Barry's house in Southsea, Hampshire. Then I drove down and helped pack up a lifetime of belongings and took Dad to his new home.

Dad loved the idea of living near the coast. He'd loved the sea ever since his time in the Royal Navy. Each day he would get up and go for walks so he could see the waves rolling in and feel the wind and sea spray on his face – he was happy there. And for me it was far better too as I could drive down from London to see him in under a couple of hours. The warden was wonderful and it was a huge relief to know there were always people around to keep an eye on him and make sure he was eating and looking after himself.

Dad's illness had progressed quite quickly and his memory was not good, but totally unlike Mum's experience, his general mood and approach to life improved as his Alzheimer's worsened. He found speaking difficult, which was frustrating for him, but he would smile and laugh when we were together – it was such a relief that he didn't carry the same sadness and depression as Mum had when she was ill. It was also nice to spend time with him when for so many years our relationship had been strained because of my anger that he had abdicated responsibility for so much of Mum's care.

David and Andrew would visit regularly as well and carers went in three times a day to check he was OK. But his behaviour became increasingly erratic as the months passed by. Once I arrived and his pants were hanging off a lampshade. Another time he dropped his trousers in the front room.

'Dad! I don't want to see that!' I laughed – and he was laughing too.

This was a man who would never even let us see him without a shirt on when we were kids. He had changed so much, but I was unbelievably relieved that this time the disease hadn't caused the terrible sadness and fear that it did for Mum. And he was also able to live a fairly independent life, though there were times when he went out and then, feeling confused, forgot how to get home. I made him little cards with his name and address on, which he could hand to people if he got lost, but I'm not sure they really helped. Once he had become lost and agitated, he would never think to find the cards and hand them over to a stranger. I just had to hope and trust that most people are good-hearted and would guide him home if he became lost.

Often I'd get a call from the warden of the complex saying Dad had gone missing and the police had been called to look for him. It was always utterly terrifying. I'd jump in my old Mini and hurtle down to Southsea with my mind on overdrive, thinking of all the awful things that could have happened to him.

Because I had spoken openly about my family's experience with Alzheimer's disease in the past, I was contacted in 2009 by a Channel 4 *Dispatches* documentary team to film a programme on the subject. Although it was painful discussing how Alzheimer's had impacted our family, I felt it was important to use my public profile to raise awareness of what it was like for families living with it. What I loved about the *Dispatches* show was that I would be meeting other families who were also struggling with Alzheimer's – I felt there was a desperate need for greater support for them.

I was very proud of the finished programme – *Mum, Dad, Alzheimer's & Me*. My brothers were also pleased that Dad's illness could help other families who were suffering. We filmed some of it in Dad's flat in Southsea. There are clips of me and him going through an old photo album. In one of the clips I am pointing at a picture of me holding Nat when he was still a baby and I say, 'Do you know who that is, Dad?' He looks at the picture but is very confused and says, 'Goodness me! I've just seen it and said it and it goes again.'

I had to explain it was me.

It is such a tender moment between us. It is then I remember him as my lovely dad. When I see him in the documentary looking so vulnerable, it is hard to accept I now have the condition he had then.

We had an incredible response from viewers to that documentary. There were thousands of emails and letters from viewers and it was a stark reminder to me of how many people in Britain were struggling with Alzheimer's, with very little support and no hope that things were ever likely to improve for them.

Within weeks of the show being aired, *Dispatches* came back to me, saying there was a huge demand for a follow-up. Quickly, we began work on another programme, which was called *My Family and Alzheimer's* and aired the following year, 2010. In that documentary, we investigated whether there had been any improvements in financial support and respite care for families but, of course, there hadn't. If anything, things seemed to be getting worse for those coping with the disease. By then the new Conservative government had begun its programme of austerity, which followed the economic crash. All sorts of public services were being cut. And Alzheimer's – which still had the image of being about old people who were going to die soon anyway – always seemed to be at the bottom of government priorities.

It seemed to me that proper funding into Alzheimer's

research and well-resourced respite care for families caring for someone with the illness were essential. The number of people living longer and getting the illness was going up and up, and without a proper strategy to try to tackle it and care for the carers, costs would only balloon for the whole of society.

Dad continued muddling along in the best way he could. I was grateful I was able to spend more time with him and we had great times together. We'd go out for lunch down by the sea or go for a wander around the town. He was still able to walk well and loved getting out and about.

Since he'd developed Alzheimer's, Dad had rediscovered a love of music that he'd lost in the middle of his life when he spent years angry about how things had turned out for him. Quite often people with the illness can remember song lyrics from years ago even when they can't remember anything from recent events. And that was Dad. So, whenever I went to visit him, we would have a bit of a sing-song or dance the way Mum and Dad had danced that night they met in north Wales.

His favourite song was Patsy Cline's 'Crazy'. One afternoon we were dancing around his front room to that. It got to the bit where Patsy sings 'I'm crazy' and Dad laughed, 'I *am* bloody crazy!' It was very funny – and so sweet.

In those final years I always felt happy when I was with him. He was funny and warm with me. And when I left to drive home I'd feel OK because he seemed happy in himself despite everything that was going on. I wasn't weighed down with guilt in the same way I had been with Mum.

Not working all the time meant I was also able to spend more time with the boys too, whether they liked it or not! And around that time Mackenzie did need me. He had always been a sensitive child who worried about things more than his older brother and like a lot of kids, he went through a terrible phase where he simply wouldn't go to school.

Every Monday, he would point-blank refuse to leave the house. Tuesdays to Friday were fine, but at the start of the week he couldn't face it. I tried everything. I'd beg him to go in, if only for ten minutes, just to get him through the door. Other times I'd be shouting at him that he didn't have a choice, he had to go. I tried bribery, I tried everything, but nothing would sway him. I spent hours trying to talk to him about how he was feeling and what was causing his sense of anxiety: was it bullying? Was it the pressure of work? Was there anything we could do to alleviate the anxiety? He couldn't fully explain what he was feeling – the thought of school on a Monday morning was just too overwhelming for him. It made for incredibly high tensions in the house at the start of every week. From lunch-time on Sunday, I would be dreading it.

We even took him to clinical psychologists who gave him coping mechanisms to manage his anxiety, but that didn't work. And the school tried to encourage him, but that was no good either. Then one Monday I managed to get him in the car and delivered him to school. I felt if we could just break the habit, maybe he'd be OK. But Mackenzie was so frustrated and angry by that point that he lashed out at the deputy headmaster – it was just awful. I was mortified and so angry at what he had done, but I could see too that he was really struggling. He wasn't a naughty boy and he didn't want to be behaving like this, he was like a cornered animal.

This went on for months and months and in the end, we took him to see the Speakmans – the celebrity life-change experts who often appear on television. Nik and Eva Speakman believe that all bad habits are due to something that has happened in our past and they help people work out what that is and how to manage it. I don't know exactly how they did it but, within a couple of sessions, Mackenzie was a totally changed child. They taught him how to manage his anxieties and from then on, he was able to cope with school again – even on a Monday morning. It was an enormous relief.

I wanted to be around for the boys when they were going through difficult times at school because I felt guilty I hadn't always been there for them when they were younger. But just when I was trying my hardest to be a good mum, there were a couple of paparazzi who earned a small fortune trying to get the right shot of me looking like an entirely frazzled mum on the school run. The thing is, I already knew I could look like a down and out in the morning! Now I didn't have to get up so early any more, often I wouldn't go to bed until 1 a.m., but that meant I wasn't looking like Elle Macpherson when I dropped the boys off at school. Who does? I'd have clean teeth and a clean face, but that was it.

So they would take these awful pictures of me and then put them on the front pages of women's magazines and write awful things, saying I couldn't get work and that we were being forced to sell our house. In the school playground, other mothers would come up to me, concerned, and ask, 'Are you all right?'

I really didn't need that kind of publicity when I was trying to do new work and enjoy my life again. And, while I knew the stuff they were writing was absolute rubbish, it did have an impact on me.

Years earlier, I'd have been furious and up for the fight with whoever was publishing such nonsense, but then it just fuelled my insecurity. I started thinking, *Oh God, what if they're right? What if I do never work again?*

Things were changing for Martin's career then too.

In 2010, ITV bought the breakfast show franchise and kicked out *GMTV*, which meant he and all the people he'd been working with lost their jobs. It came as a massive shock to him. I'd been defined by my job when I was on breakfast TV, but Martin was a full-on workaholic. And as an editor he didn't think there would be many other jobs open to him. It was a huge blow to his sense of identity and didn't make relations in our marriage any easier. I knew I'd been difficult to live with for a fair while, but that was a bad patch for him too.

There were stories in the newspapers that our marriage was at breaking point. I don't think we were in more of a crisis than anyone else's marriage goes through at times, but it was bumpy. It was hard for Martin. I think deep down men still believe they're hunter-gatherers and being made redundant is a huge dent to their pride.

After a couple of months of moping around, Martin realized

he'd had enough of the whole London TV scene and decided what he needed was 'A Change'.

'How about a pub?' he said one night.

'A what?!'

'A pub – I could buy a pub in Dorset. We love Dorset and the boys are happy there. And let's be honest, I only know two things – journalism and how to enjoy a glass of wine. If the journalism is over, it must be time to try the wine option. And I've got my redundancy money, which would be enough to get us going – it could be a new start.'

To me it sounded like a classic male mid-life crisis – successful TV executive loses job and then ploughs every spare penny into a dream that will inevitably crash and burn.

What's not to like?

Martin always says I'm the most stubborn person he's ever met, but he's pretty determined himself too. I knew if that was what he had set his sights on, there was little point in arguing.

We loved Dorset and had spent lots of time down there over the past few years. It always felt like an escape from London and it was only a two and a half hours' drive from our house. In fact, we loved it so much that a couple of years earlier, we had bought ourselves a little holiday home in a village near the coast. Martin started looking near there for the perfect pub and within a short amount of time we were the proud owners of The Greyhound Inn, a gastropub with a few rooms upstairs.

The plan was that at first Martin would commute back and forwards a couple of times a week while I stayed in London with the boys. In the longer term, who knew? If it worked, maybe at some point we'd all move down there. Part of me was excited about the new adventure. Remember, my grandad and grandma had run the pub in Canterbury so I did have some idea what we were getting ourselves into. And I liked the idea that after years of us both being at the mercy of the broadcasting industry, where your face can fit one day and not the next, we would have some-thing that was completely ours, although we never planned to become the Bet Lynch and Alec Gilroy of Dorset. The intention was to employ managers to run the place on a day-to-day basis.

At first it worked really well. I would often go down at weekends with the boys and we'd have great times. But as the boys got older with their own friends and activities – not to mention their obsession with Chelsea F.C. – they were less enthusiastic about travelling to Dorset every weekend. And I started to get fed up with it all a bit too. There's a huge amount of work running a pub and so whenever me and the boys went down there, we would barely see Martin as he was hard at it, either serving behind the bar, dealing with guests or trying to work out staffing rotas.

It became incredibly stressful, trying to find good chefs and managers, and a lot of time was spent dealing with customers' questions and gripes. And with Martin away most of the week it all just added to my sense that everything at home got left to me. If I wasn't there looking after the boys, keeping the house tidy, cleaning football boots, putting the bins out, filling in all those endless forms that schools send home and all the other stuff of family life then it wouldn't have got done. And

I did start to resent that. Of course all that just led to more rows as Martin was working every hour God sends down in Dorset and when he did come home, he'd get an earful from me! Then about a year after Martin bought the pub, it got broken into.

It felt like everything was falling apart.

While I was doing all the hard yards at home, I was still trying to work as much as I could too. I was still writing my weekly column for the *Daily Mirror*, hosting a radio show for Magic FM and presenting *OK!TV*, as well as creating a string of one-off documentaries. I even appeared on ITV's *Loose Women* a couple of times. I hated it, though – I really wasn't comfortable on a show where the whole point was airing your dirty laundry in public. Mum would have been horrified! I don't mind a good gossip in private, but I felt very uncomfortable doing it in public. Sometimes I would stand in on the *Lorraine* show when Lorraine Kelly was on holiday and that was fun because I did miss the adrenaline rush of live television.

Despite having a calmer life, the black cloud that seemed to have been hanging over me leading to this sense of listlessness and weight never entirely lifted. I suppose, in hindsight, I still hadn't really shifted the depression that had hit me during my final years at *GMTV*. Perhaps I knew that on one level, but I didn't want to entirely accept it. I wasn't one of those people who was going to lie on a couch telling a therapist about my life – and I certainly wasn't going to start popping pills containing God knows what to make me feel better! I just hoped in time I'd get over the incredible sadness that I still felt about Mum and Dad, that life at home would become a bit easier and maybe, just maybe, I could return to my old self.

15

What happened to my dad in the three months between the end of 2011 and his death in February the following year is one of the experiences that stays with me most when I think about Alzheimer's. I talk a lot now about how my poor dad suffered in his final months and days. Is that because I'm scared one day it could happen to me? Maybe.

It was truly terrifying to see how people can be treated when they have our disease (it is 'our disease' now – a Phillips family heirloom!). Despite being very confused and struggling to even recognize his family at times, Dad had managed to continue a reasonable life in Southsea. There would be times I would go to visit and there was only a flicker of recognition in his eyes, but he remained in good spirits and would tell rambling, funny stories, laughing along to himself. It was such a far cry from all those years when he'd seemed so angry at the world. But then quite near Christmas 2011, I got a call one afternoon from the warden at the complex where he lived.

'Hi, Fiona, I'm really sorry,' she said, 'but it's your dad. He's not in his flat and we think he must have wandered off again. The police are out looking for him.'

The temperature was falling below freezing and I was terrified if he wasn't found quickly, he would be dead from exposure before the morning. He'd lost a lot of weight in recent years and was pretty much skin and bone – he wouldn't survive a frosty night. Or maybe he would walk out into the sea or get hit by a car and if he wasn't carrying any identification, we might never find him. I was frantic with worry.

He was missing for eight hours before the police finally got a call from a casino in nearby Portsmouth to say a man was acting strangely. It was Dad. Goodness only knows how he ended up there, but he was utterly confused. Social services had to be informed and they said Dad couldn't go back to his flat alone. Apparently, it wouldn't be safe so he would have to go straight to a specialist dementia care home to be checked out. I had known that the time would come when he would need to be looked after in a care home, but I'd been putting that off for as long as possible. Independence meant everything to my dad and even in his most confused state I knew he would hate being surrounded by people fussing over him.

But it seemed like that time had definitely come. And while I knew he wouldn't like it, I also felt a strange sense of relief. The decision had been taken away from me and I could be reassured he would be getting properly looked after by people trained in caring for dementia.

The morning after he was admitted I went to visit him at the care home. He was still confused and didn't know who I was or what I was doing there, but he seemed happy enough. Maybe at that point though he didn't realize this wasn't just a brief visit to the home – this was where he was going to be living from then on.

It was only twenty-four hours later when I received a call from the home to say Dad's mood had totally changed. Something had happened that had upset him and he had lashed out at a member of staff. Obviously, I didn't want my dad to be frightening people, but I could see how it might have happened – I had hoped the staff might be a bit more under-standing. He was in an entirely strange place, surrounded by people he didn't know; he was unable to speak properly and had no other way of expressing his anxiety and confusion. So, like a child, he lashed out. I tried to calm Dad down and pleaded with him to just go along with things for the time being, but he was clearly very agitated.

The following night he became even more angry and distressed and grabbed hold of another resident around the neck and was shouting abuse at the television. The manager of the home was straight back on the phone to me. They said they couldn't cope and it was too distressing for other residents – he would have to leave. I couldn't believe they were kicking an old, seriously ill and very confused man out on his ear, but they weren't budging. I was furious. After all the upheaval of getting him into the home, he'd now be sent to another new and bewil-dering place.

But it was to get far worse. Rather than being transferred to another care home, Dad was sent to a psychiatric hospital, where he was immediately put on a mixture of powerful drugs and sedatives. I don't think I realized at first how many drugs they were pumping into him, or maybe they just took a while to kick in.

Two days before Christmas, on 23 December, I went down to visit him. I had armfuls of presents – socks and a jumper and some new slippers. There were cards from the boys for their grandad. As soon as I stepped in the room he looked up and beamed at me: 'She's mine,' he said, smiling and laughing. It had been his way of greeting me for a while. He couldn't always remember my name or exactly who I was, but he knew I was his – which I always was.

I chatted with the members of staff and everyone was talking about getting ready for Christmas and it was a lovely day. When I returned just a few days after the Christmas break, Dad had changed beyond all recognition. As I walked into the room, he didn't even look up. There was no 'she's mine' and a hearty laugh. He was slumped in his chair, clearly off his head on all the drugs they must have used to sedate him.

I sat down right next to him to look into his eyes, but he couldn't focus on me at all – he was looking through me to another world. And when I looked in his eyes, it truly felt like my dad was gone. His soul had been entirely erased by whatever drugs they'd been pumping into him. I held his hand and rubbed his fingers, desperately trying to bring him back to his senses so he could at least be aware that I was there, but he was too far gone.

I could feel anger rising up in front of me. In the space of a handful of days over Christmas while Dad had been in that place they'd stolen his soul. That was what it felt like.

I went to see the duty nurse and asked to see what drugs they'd been giving him. She scurried off and returned a short time afterwards with a clipboard on which two entire sides of A4 paper were covered in the names of different medication they'd been administering to him over the past few days.

'This is way too much,' I said, trying not to explode with rage. 'He's like a zombie over there with the amount that you're giving him. You have got to reduce it. Immediately.'

Of course they didn't want to reduce any of the medication. So often people in authority just think they know best, but I knew my dad and this wasn't best for him. I was not going to be talked around and, after much debate, they agreed to lower the amount of one of his sedatives.

I stayed with him for the rest of the day and tried to get him out of the chair to move around, but he struggled to stand up and remained stooped over, shuffling across the room. This was a man who only days earlier had walked around the town for eight hours before turning up at a casino. Obviously, he shouldn't have been doing that, but it showed how he was still physically able. Now he could barely put one foot in front of the other.

After I left Dad that night, I drove straight home to London and began googling all the medication on the list to find out what on earth they had been pumping into him. I felt sick when I saw the effects of some of those drugs. Two of the sedatives were highly addictive and were found to cause cognitive decline and the anti-psychotic they had put him on was only supposed to be used as a last resort and was known to increase the risk of death in those with dementia. All the reports I read explained Dad's stooped and shuffling walk was a classic symptom of someone heavily medicated on such drugs.

I went back a few days later, by which time Dad's condition had deteriorated even further. The doctors claimed they had reduced some of his medication, but they refused to withdraw it altogether. I felt I had no choice but to go along with the 'experts' – I hated it.

Within a really short space of time, the medication made Dad put on weight and appear bloated, while his hair turned almost entirely white. One morning I walked in and barely recognized the old man sitting in an armchair.

'Oh, Dad,' I said, 'what have they done to you?' And I broke down in tears. But there was no response from my dad, he couldn't comfort me. He couldn't do anything by then, he was totally out of it – his body had been clobbered with drugs.

And things only got worse. From then on, whenever I visited him he was like someone out of *One Flew Over the Cuckoo's Nest* – totally out of it. And then, on one visit, it was even worse. His eyes were glazed, his mouth was hanging open and his tongue was lolling. It was heartbreaking.

If I picked up his hand then let go, it would drop down like a rock – he had no control over his limbs. His eyes were opaque and watering, unable to focus on anything. He was there, but not really there.

I was backwards and forwards several times a week. On one

visit as soon as I sat down and held his hand I could tell he was very warm. I put my palm across his forehead, like I used to do with the boys when they were little, and I could instantly feel he had a temperature. His breathing didn't sound quite right to me either. It was laboured as though he was trying to catch enough air for his lungs. How long had he been like this and why on earth had none of the nurses noticed?

I'm sure the hospital staff felt I was constantly complaining about the way Dad was being looked after, but I didn't care what they thought. He was my dad and I wanted the best for him. They said they'd keep a closer eye on him over the next few days and maybe they did, but six days later, on a Thursday, he was admitted to a general hospital with pneumonia. I shot straight down to the hospital in Gosport and found him on a ward looking incredibly poorly. His eyes were closed and any colour had gone from his face.

After I got there, the doctor caring for him came over and sat down next to me. I knew this was bad news – the worst news.

'I'm afraid your father is very ill,' he said. 'His kidneys are no longer functioning properly and his organs are failing, but we are of course trying to do whatever we can for him.'

Even then, crazily, I thought things might be all right. I thought that lovely doctor would manage to bring him back from the brink.

'We'll get you out of that awful unit and find you a beautiful new home where you'll he happy,' I told Dad as he lay there, eyes closed and sleeping. 'We'll get those awful drugs out of your system and you'll be back to your funny old self – but no more casinos for you!'

I spent all that weekend with Dad but, as it got closer to Monday, I started to realize I was fooling myself: Dad was only getting weaker. My brothers came down and spent time with him too and we chatted around his bed, hoping that maybe he could hear us even though he appeared fast asleep. I massaged his neck and stroked his hand and we told stories about when we were young – about Rufus the bonkers dog and all the days we'd spent sitting on the beach in Wales in the pouring rain.

I was still there on the Tuesday and knew Dad was slipping from us, which was why I was determined to stay. David and I had been sitting at his bed, but in the afternoon we decided to pop out quickly for a coffee and some fresh air. When we returned an hour later there was a line of staff ushering us into a room, where one of the nurses said, 'I'm so sorry, your dad has gone.'

It seemed too much to take in. Dad, who'd been distant when we were kids, had been so present in our lives in recent years even as the real essence of who he was had slipped further away. Now he was gone entirely.

David and I asked to see him. We went to his bedside and he looked so peaceful. I held his hand and kissed him.

I drove home to London, barely able to see the road for the tears in my eyes. Now I knew what it was to have no mum or dad. I had my lovely boys and Martin, but I felt very alone at that point and I was angry too – angry, as I didn't think Dad should be dead. Yes, he'd been poorly with Alzheimer's, but physically he'd still been fit and he was happy and content until they'd stuffed him full of those drugs. I felt that because he'd had Alzheimer's, some of the medics hadn't thought it really mattered if he lived or died or if he was pumped to the eyeballs with sedatives. Would they have done that to a younger person or someone who was agitated but didn't have Alzheimer's? I don't think so. They hadn't understood that he was still a person in his own right, who was still giving so much to me and my brothers just by being there. We didn't want him so sedated. It crushed his soul – and he most certainly wouldn't have wanted that either.

A couple of weeks later, we had Dad's funeral. My brothers and all the extended family were there and it was a lovely goodbye for him. I'd asked for them to play Patsy Cline's 'Crazy' as one of the pieces of music – when it started up on the speaker, I was inconsolable. It was grief but also fury that Dad had been taken from us. He shouldn't have gone. Not then. If he hadn't been given those drugs, he could still have been there, still laughing, still dancing. Of course his mind wasn't coming back, but he could still have been happy.

It broke my heart all over again.

16

Martin

———————

I felt it might be a good moment for me to reappear to talk about how I recall those years when Fiona was going through so much. I know it may be unusual in a book to have a different voice chipping in every now and again – I wonder how different all autobiographies would be if family and friends were included intermittently to lend alternative perspectives on certain events.

As Fiona has said, Amy's illness had a terrible impact on her. It was just so exhausting, all that driving backwards and forwards to Wales. On top of the emotional impact of seeing her mum slipping away from her, I think she was caught up in a vicious circle of trying to do everything she could to care for her, but always feeling it wasn't enough. Of course, she had two little boys to look after, as well as an incredibly demanding job.

Sometimes I'd try to suggest that she was putting too much stress on herself – and our entire family – but that rarely ended well. If Fiona had an idea in her head there was absolutely no point in trying to talk her out of it. She very firmly felt it was her responsibility to care for her mum however she could and nothing was going to stand in the way of that.

Amy was poorly from the time I met Fiona so I never knew the bright, vivacious woman that she spoke about although occasionally there would be glimpses of what she must have been like years before. For me, I just saw a woman who seemed desperately frightened and lonely. I totally understand why Fiona felt compelled to do everything she could to comfort her, but I think it came at a terrible personal cost to her – she was constantly shattered. But I too was a workaholic, we were both very driven people – we just got on with stuff.

Soon after her mum's death, her dad – Phil – was diagnosed with the same condition, so a lot of Fiona's attention transferred to worrying about him and travelling back and forth to Southsea. The rest of the time we were in that routine of life that most people have – working, looking after the kids and going out or seeing our friends whenever we had any energy left to do so.

And then, in 2008, Fiona left *GMTV*. It was a massive knock to her pride and confidence. Fiona really doesn't have a big ego, unlike so many people in the world of TV, but it was still a jolt. Yes, she had found the job tough when she had two young children and was making those constant trips back and forth to Wales to care for her parents, but she did it. And she was incredibly good at it. Guests loved her and she had a way of connecting with interviewees, be they celebrities or ordinary people, which very few presenters have.

Television can be a brutal world and things keep changing. If a new boss comes in and wants to shake up the format then that's what happens – there's not really very much that a presenter can do about that. But work was – and still is – a huge part of who Fiona is. Even now, when she has become quite poorly and cannot remember so much of her life, she will frequently tell people that she was working from the age of eleven on her paper round – that incredibly strong work ethic she inherited from her dad has never left her.

When she left *GMTV* it was tough because she wanted to work even though I think even she would accept that she deserved a bit of a break after the previous few years. She put a very brave face on things and never let the public know what she truly felt – and she got on with finding more work in the freelance world. That is incredibly hard because you are having to fight for every commission, but she did get offered a lot of jobs and really enjoyed them.

She made those brilliant documentaries for *Dispatches* and *Panorama* and she is still very proud of them. Perhaps prouder of them than anything she did on breakfast television because in the world of TV you're accepted by the great and the good for that kind of work – many insiders still judge daytime TV as a lesser thing.

I suppose, like all of us, Fiona wanted to be accepted as a 'proper journalist' so the opportunity to do some hard-hitting documentaries appealed to her. That was why she was so proud of her *Mirror* column too.

Fiona may not have been earning the sums of money other TV presenters were making, but she didn't care about that. She has never been bothered about money or been one of those people who would say: 'I must have this' or 'I want to buy that'. It wasn't the money that drove her, it was the work. But after a while there were fewer freelance jobs coming around and she wasn't working as much. There were still things for her to do each day – and she spent a lot of time on her *Mirror* column – but I suppose she missed the adrenaline of presenting a daily show.

Fiona never really had any hobbies and she didn't surround herself with showbiz friends. She had a few friends locally, who she had met through having children, but mostly her life was filled with work and family. When she was at home in London, if she wasn't working she wanted to be with the boys. So, when work stopped or became more infrequent, she had a lot of time on her hands. At first she started doing up the house, buying new blinds or carpets and having sofas reupholstered even if they didn't really need to be – it filled her day but wasn't really a purpose.

We had bought a little house in Italy a few years earlier and had a holiday home in Dorset so there were always things for her to do, but she didn't love that kind of pottering around in the way that she loved work. As she has said, during that time Fiona spent a lot of time with her dad. She went down to see him every weekend or even during the week when she could, often taking the boys with her. To this day, Mackenzie still has a pathological loathing of Portsmouth! He hated the journey and was too little to understand why his grandad was acting so strangely when they got there. But Fiona really wanted to be there for her dad – she idolized him. So, when Phil passed away, that was incredibly hard for her and she was left with the anger that he had been cheated of his final months – and that sat heavily with her.

During that period, I was down in Dorset at the pub a lot of the time. I managed to keep the pub going for three years, but by the end it was losing money and I realized I had to get out. I was also getting itchy feet and wanted a way back into journalism so I started to do some freelance work for Channel 7's *Sunrise* programme, which is the biggest breakfast show in Australia. I began reporting for them from London, which meant driving up from Dorset four or five nights a week to be on air at 11 p.m. UK time in the studio. Then I'd stay overnight at home before driving back down to Dorset again the next day to check Mr and Mrs So-and-So out of Room 6.

So that was all quite stressful for our relationship too.

There wasn't time to discuss how either of us was feeling about how life and our marriage was going; we were just surviving. But that's what relationships are 90 per cent of the time – just getting through the day. During your mid-fifties, there's a sense of thinking, *Oh, is this it?* – and it kind of is. And you can just sort of muddle through, get through the day, and then it's another day.

Finally, I found a buyer for the pub and sold it in 2014, which came as a relief, but by then I had ploughed all my redundancy payout into the business and lost the lot – every penny. Being back in London was much better for the family, but there's no doubt Fiona was depressed. She had never got back into full-time TV work but, as I've said, she still enjoyed writing her *Daily Mirror* column. And she was really diligent about it, making sure she kept up with the news. She took the responsibility of writing about big events very seriously. She always wanted to do her best by the readers and she loved that it was a left-wing newspaper that shared all those values she had grown up with.

After the pub closed, I got more work in television, so it wasn't as though Fiona needed a job for the money – we had enough to get by – but she missed having a sense of purpose. I think her depression probably started when her mum was alive and she was still at *GMTV*, but when she stopped having work to focus on, it became more evident.

Could this have been the beginning of Alzheimer's? I know there are similarities with how her mum first became ill – it started with depression for her – but there was nothing else in Fiona's behaviour that seemed different. And she'd been through so much with her mum and dad and work that there were clear reasons she would be exhausted and her mental health shattered. There were plenty of times too when she could still be great fun and we'd have a great time like in the old days.

Maybe I should have really encouraged Fiona to get

treatment. Looking back, I can ask myself if I should've done more, but when you're in the middle of something like that it's almost impossible to see the bigger picture. Things weren't great, but life's not always great, is it?

17

Fiona

As Martin says, that's kind of how things continued. The boys grew up from little boys into young men who towered above me when we walked down the street (I was constantly restocking the fridge, so it must have been all that food!). And Martin's career got back on track. In 2014, he took over at ITV's *Loose Women* and, after a spell sorting that out, he became editor of *This Morning* with Phillip Schofield and Holly Willoughby the following year. Things were going great for him – he was back where he wanted to be, in the heart of the TV action.

As for me, bits and pieces of work came in over the years that followed, but I never felt completely right. Was I worried that there might be something sinister lurking beneath the surface? That Alzheimer's could one day be coming for me too?

Soon after Dad died in February 2012, I did an interview with Alison Phillips (no relation, but she is now helping me write this book!). Back then, she was an editor and columnist at the *Daily Mirror*. We met in a hotel in west London and I soon found myself being way more open than I had intended to be – but then that's me.

'I think the clock is ticking,' I said. 'I think Alzheimer's has taken Mum and Dad and it's now only a matter of time before it will come for me.'

It seemed all too likely that if my parents had suffered in this way, there was a pretty strong chance that I would be impacted one day. Alison asked how that made me feel – whether I was angry or scared about it. At that point, maybe because I'd been feeling so low, I had almost resigned myself to it.

'I keep thinking I might only have five years left,' I said. 'But it's making me think I'd better make the most of life, so that's positive, I suppose.

'I feel I've got to do everything now in case my mind goes. So often I've thought, "I'd love to go there or see that," but I haven't because of work or something. But now if I want to do something, I just do it.'

But the strange thing was, although I could say that out loud and, on one level, I did think I would get the disease, there was also another part of me that was in a strange sort of denial about it all. It was like I was able to operate two parallel lives – one of acceptance of what might happen and another in absolute refusal. Maybe that's what was in conflict when I did become ill.

Although I could discuss my anxieties about becoming ill in an interview, I didn't do so at home. Talking to the people you love most about something like that makes it somehow more real. Instead I packed every day with activity, eager to try to cram my life with experiences and avoid thinking about things that were worrying me.

Even in the evenings, I couldn't just lie in front of the television – I'd be up dusting, plumping the curtains and cleaning the kitchen.

I had to keep busy.

Martin would say to me, 'Will you just sit down!' But I couldn't – I had to be on the go all the time.

I started doing everything recommended to keep the brain healthy. I began taking gingko biloba, a herbal medicine supposed to aid memory. And I stuck to the vegetarian diet I'd had since I was a teenager. I didn't smoke and only drank occasionally. But really, trying to hold back Alzheimer's with a healthy lifestyle is like trying to hold back the tide with a fishing net – if it's coming for you, I think that's that.

And over the months and years that followed I wasn't always consistent about whether I thought I would get the disease. Sometimes I would reject the whole idea entirely.

'This illness has devastated so much of my life already, surely it's not going to come for me too?' I'd tell friends. 'Lightning doesn't strike twice. Well, even if it does, it definitely doesn't strike three times.'

Was that wishful thinking? Maybe, but there were times I truly believed it.

Other times in interviews I would say I was terrified I would get it. I think the truth is I was often looking for things to distract myself from the idea. I couldn't face the whole prospect. Trying to unpick all this now is difficult. I find it hard to remember how I felt, but reading things I wrote at the time I was clearly worried and trying not to be overwhelmed by that.

In 2017, I was commissioned by the BBC to make a documentary called *The Truth About Stress*. During the research, I became convinced that the pressure I'd been under when I was doing *GMTV* and caring for my mum had caused chronic stress, which was still impacting me years later.

I found this whole area fascinating. I read all the scientific research that shows stress can reduce life expectancy and cause heart disease, dementia and cancer. I didn't dwell on the dementia aspect too much – that was something I really didn't want to be thinking about.

During the course of my research, what I found interesting was that stress can also be good for us as humans – it's a primal emotion that helps us fight or escape danger, so it can enhance performance. And I think for a long time that stress did help me do my job well on television. But when you're permanently stressed out and you go to bed and your stomach is still churning, when you can't sleep and every time you breathe you have that churning stomach thing going on, that's chronic stress.

When I look back at the show, I appear bright and alert – maybe even too alert. Perhaps I was then 'living on my nerves' as my mum would have said. What you don't see in a short documentary is how I was feeling the rest of the time – the way I struggled to relax and how my brain kept flitting from one thing to the other or from anxieties about the past to worries about the future. These were all classic examples of stress and how I was always trying to do a million things at the same time while thinking I hadn't done a good job of any of them.

The experts said prolonged stress could lead to anxiety and depression. The more I read about the symptoms, the more convinced I became that that's what had happened to me – my chronic stress had morphed into anxiety and depression.

But there were underlying concerns too. In one interview I did to publicize the documentary about stress, I told viewers how I was worried about my future because I kept losing my car keys. And how I went to put something in the fridge when I meant to go to the oven. Even then I was suggesting the real reason I'd lost my keys was because I was so busy and I was still half joking about it in the way people do when they say, 'Oh look, I can't remember what I'm doing – I must be going mad.' And yet beneath that I did have worries about what my future could be like, knowing as I did the awfulness of dementia and the failures in the care system.

In that interview I said I wanted to write a long letter to Martin about the future and how I would want to be looked after if I had Alzheimer's. I said I didn't want him to put me in home – which I didn't, and I still don't. But I never actually wrote that letter. Surely if I had seriously thought at that point that I might fall ill, then I would have written the letter? I really don't know. Maybe the nature of this illness is that it all happens so slowly but so constantly that it always remains one step ahead of your own understanding of what is happening.

Things between me and Martin weren't great either.

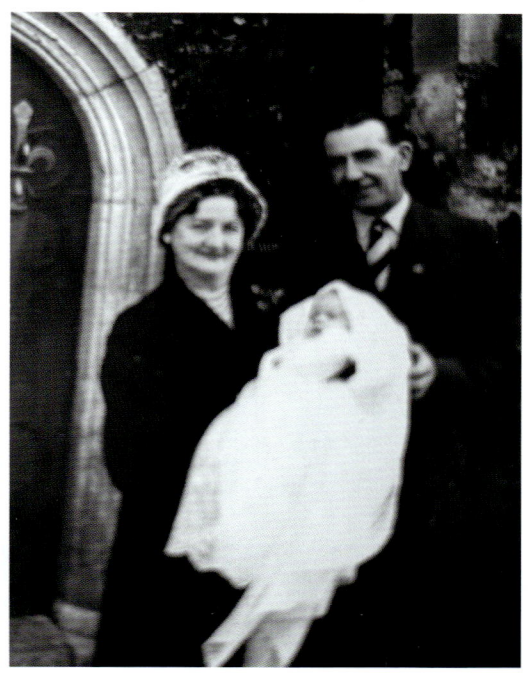

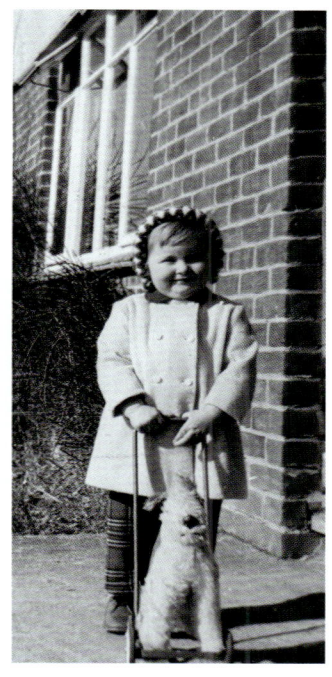

Me on my christening day at
just two months old, 1961.

Aged two, in a very fine
pair of tartan trousers!

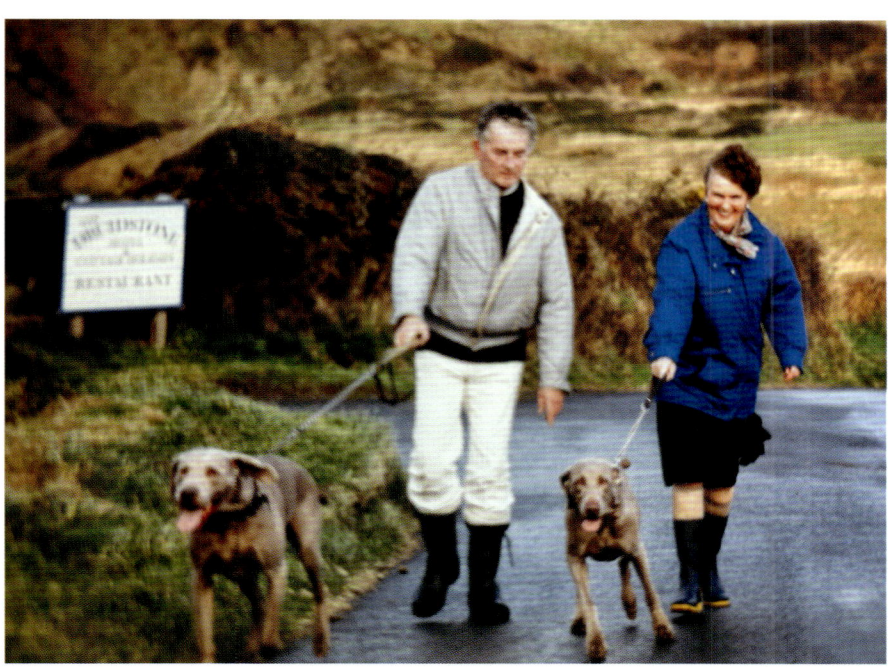

Mum smiling that wonderful smile with Dad while walking
the dogs near their home in Wales, after they moved back.

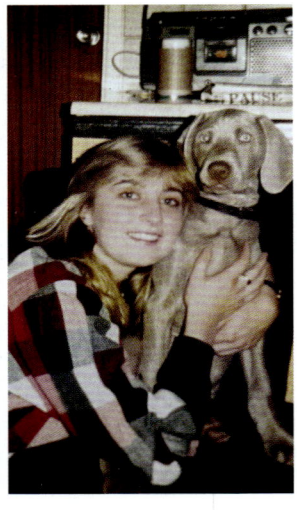

Back home from
university, aged
twenty-two.

LA days, with
Neal to my right.
Check out my
Hollywood shades!

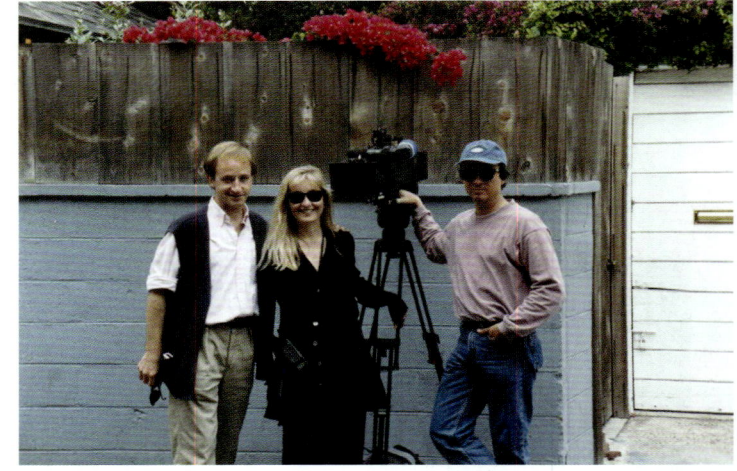

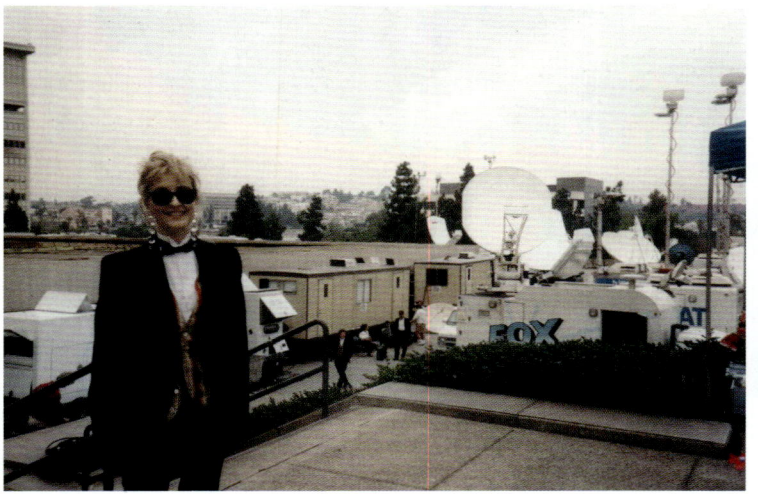

Dressed to the
nines for the
first Oscars
ceremony that
Neal and I
covered, 1993.

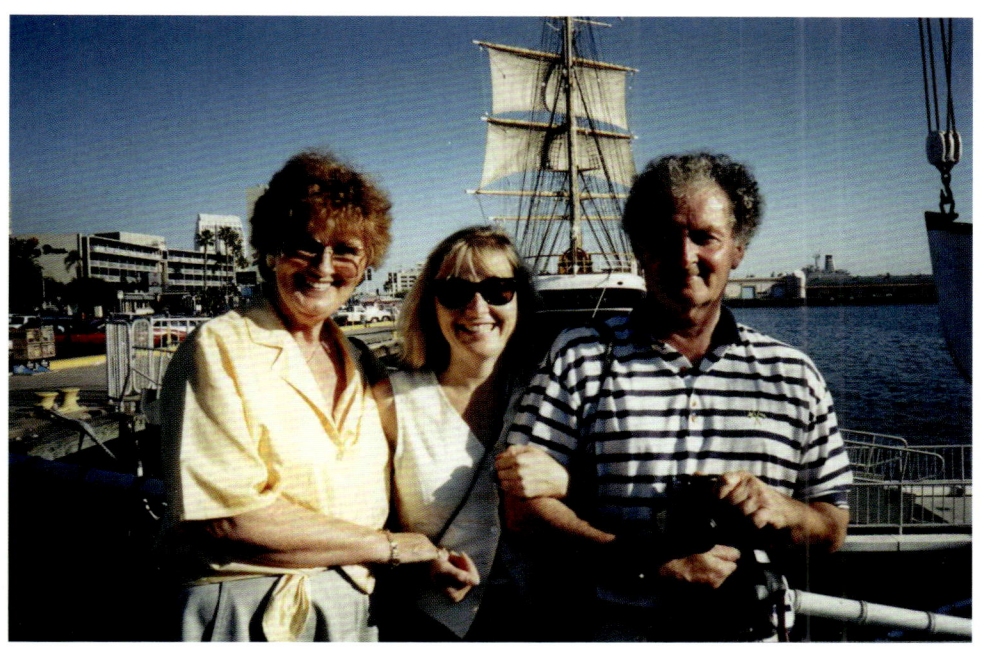

Mum and Dad's visit to LA, June 1994. Mum is smiling for the camera, but for much of that holiday she seemed distracted and depressed.

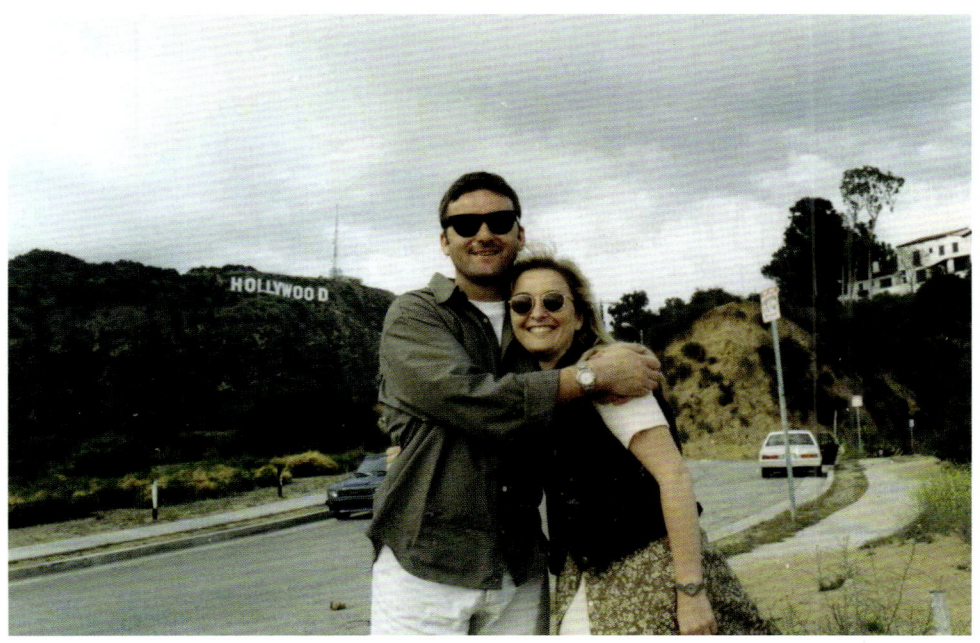

My brother David, who came out to see me in LA in 1994.

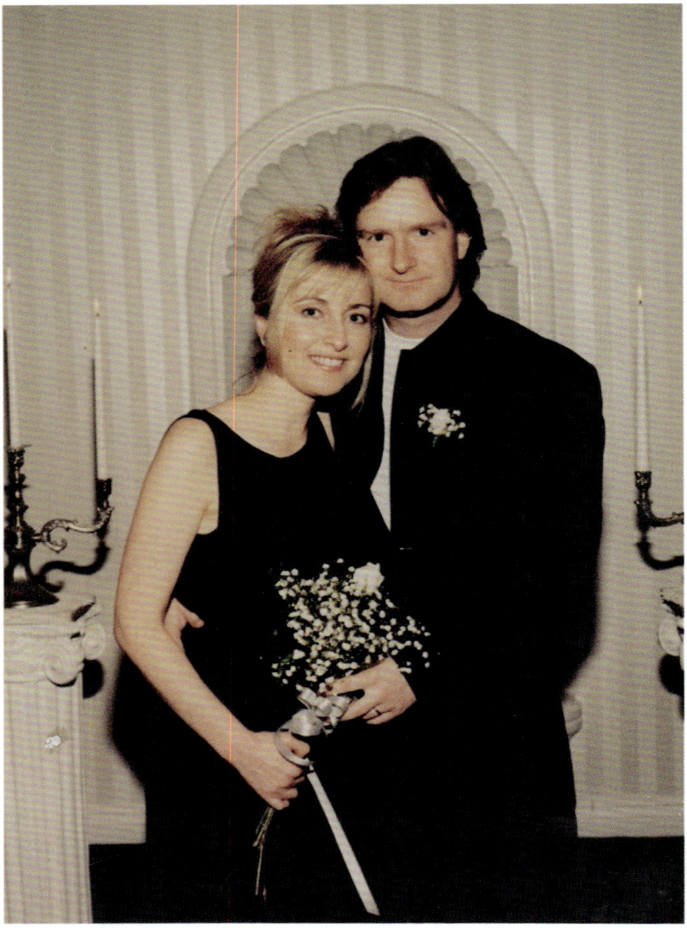

Our wonderful
wedding day,
7 May 1997, at
Little Chapel of the
Flowers in Las Vegas.

Mum with Nat,
pictured soon after
he was born in May
1999. She looks so
happy holding her
grandson, but on that
trip it was clear she
was becoming very
confused.

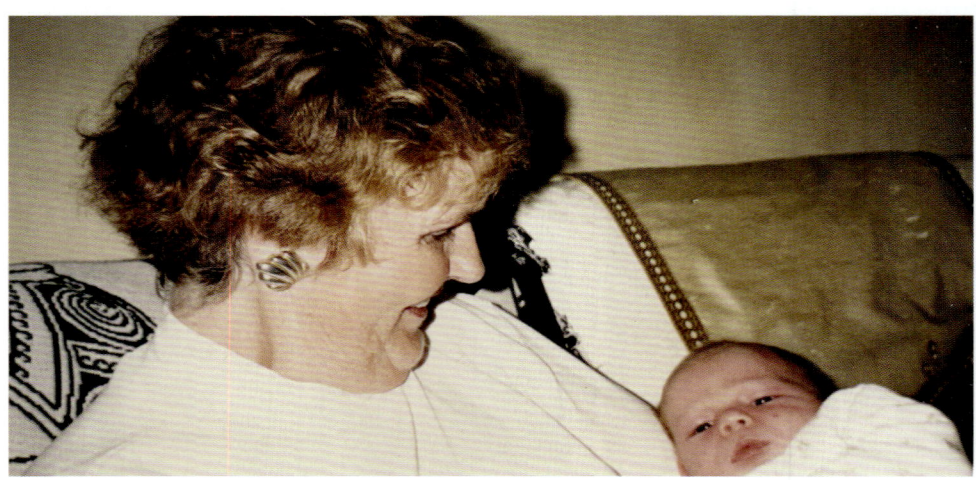

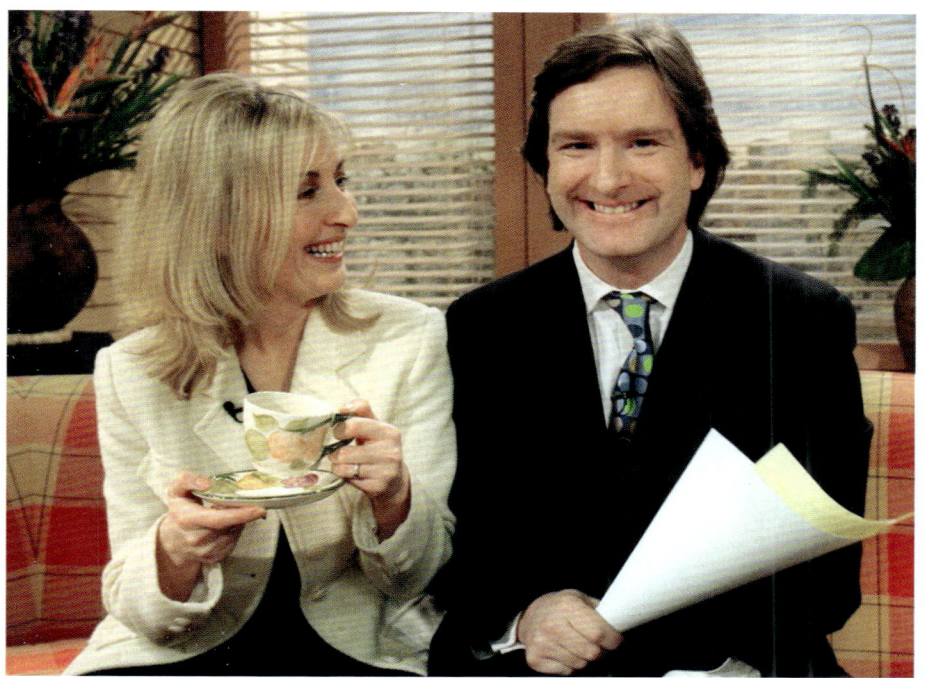

A cup of tea and a laugh with the boss – my husband, Martin –
when he became editor of *GMTV* (he knew he wasn't really the boss!).

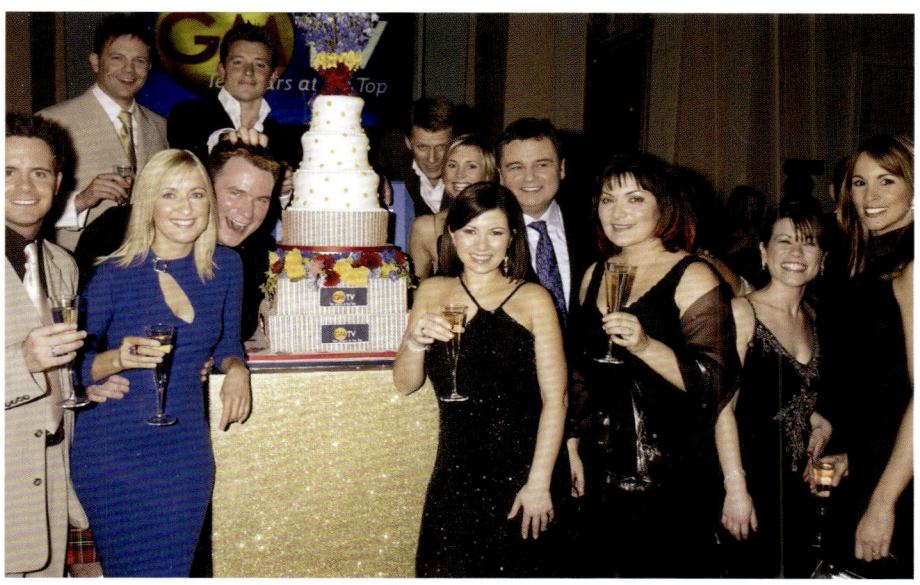

The *GMTV* tenth anniversary, 2003, with my very young-looking
colleagues, including Ben Shephard, Andrew Castle, Eamonn Holmes,
Lorraine Kelly and Andrea McLean.

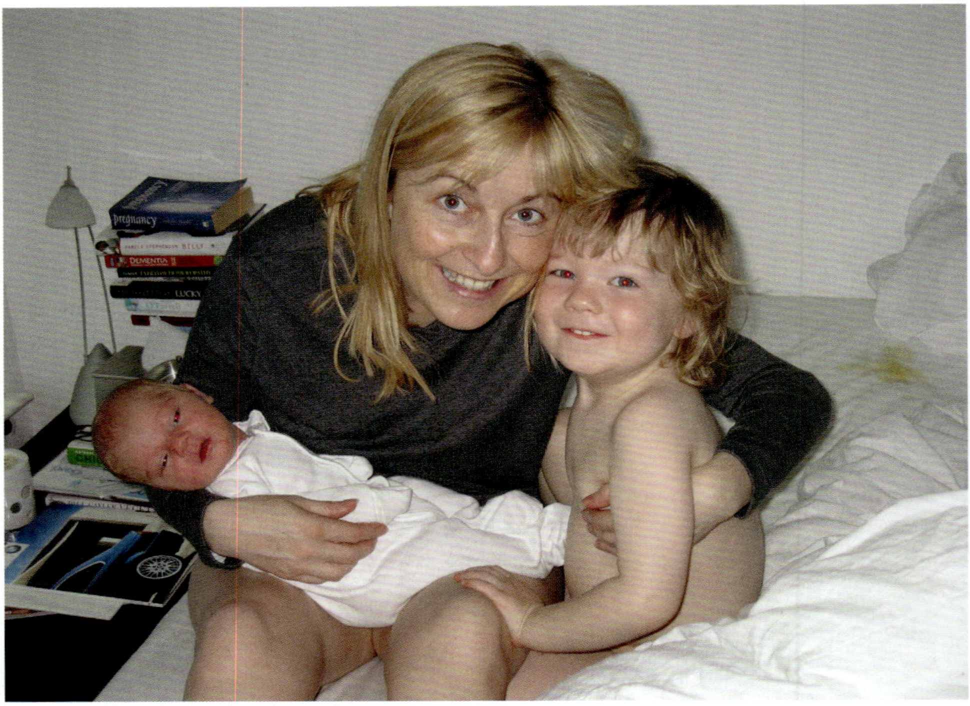

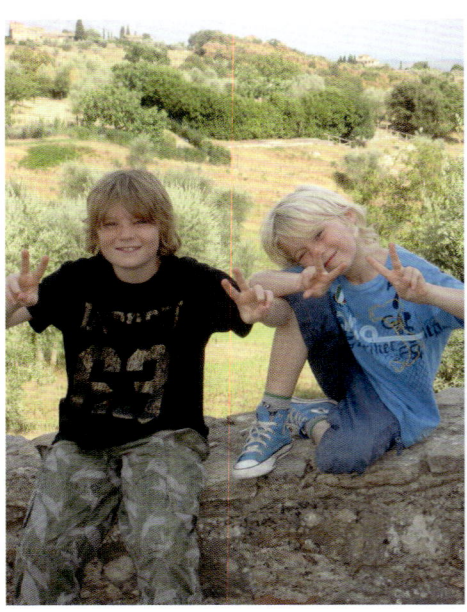

Bringing baby Mackenzie home from hospital
to meet his big brother, Nat, in May 2002.

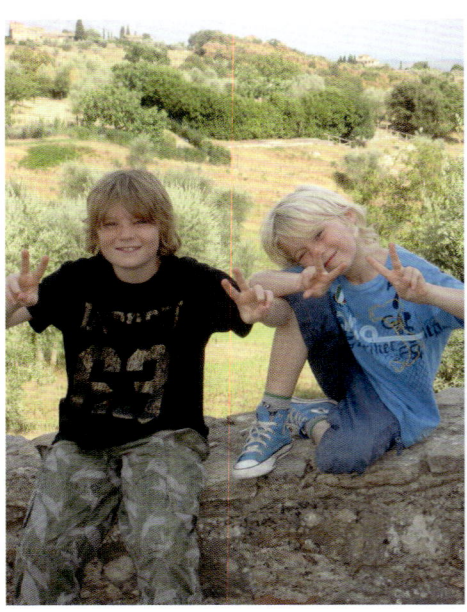

Nat and Mackenzie, as funny and
cheeky as ever on holiday in Italy.

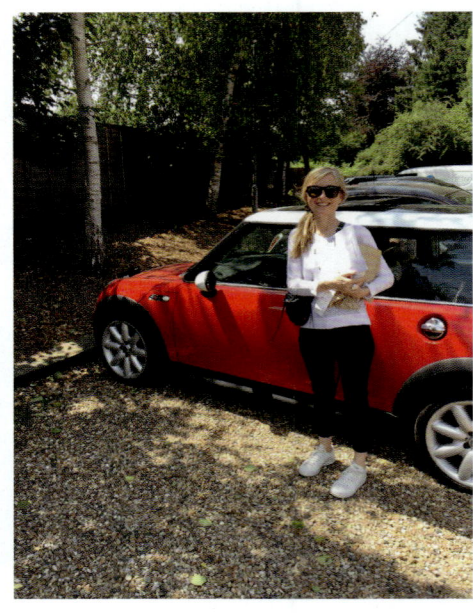

My beloved scarlet Mini Cooper,
which I drove for seventeen years.

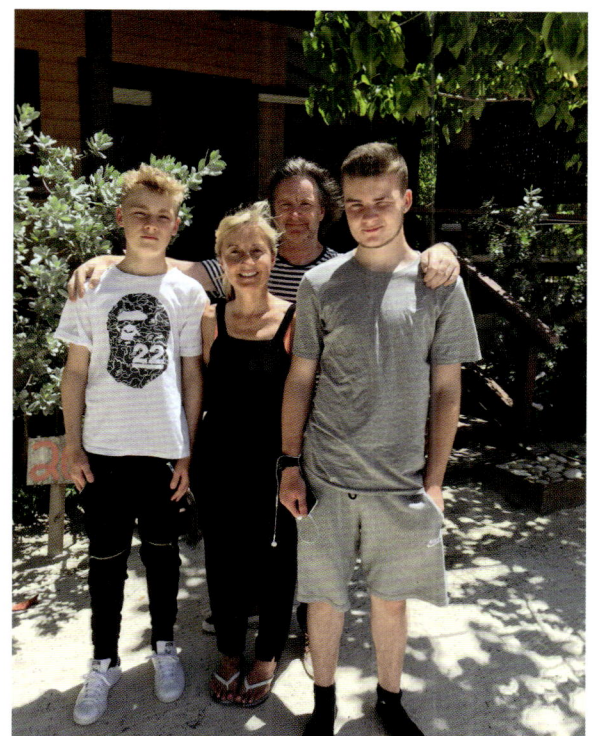

Me and my gorgeous boys on a family holiday in the Maldives.

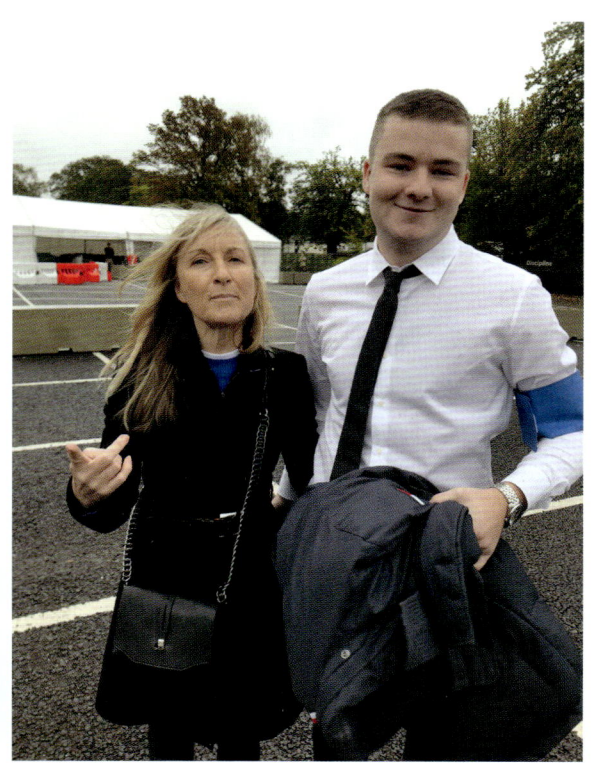

Nat's first day in the army – just as Covid was beginning in 2020.

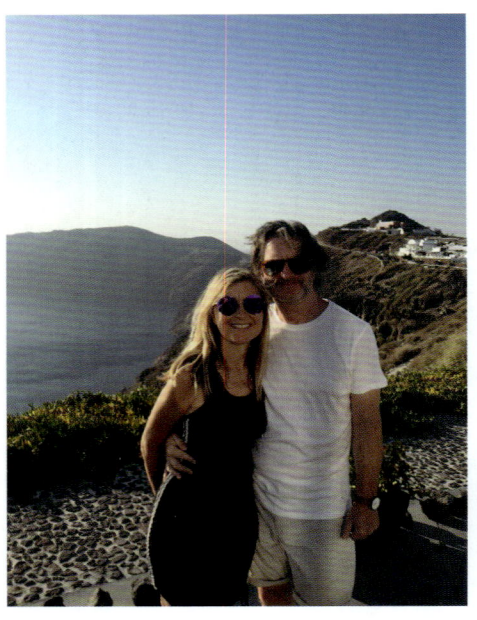

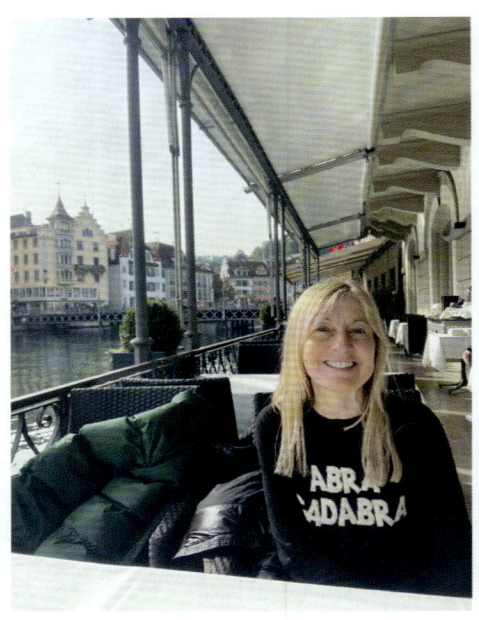

Martin and I have always enjoyed getting away together for a few days. This lovely picture was taken in Santorini.

On our trip to Lucerne, just before my Alzheimer's diagnosis.

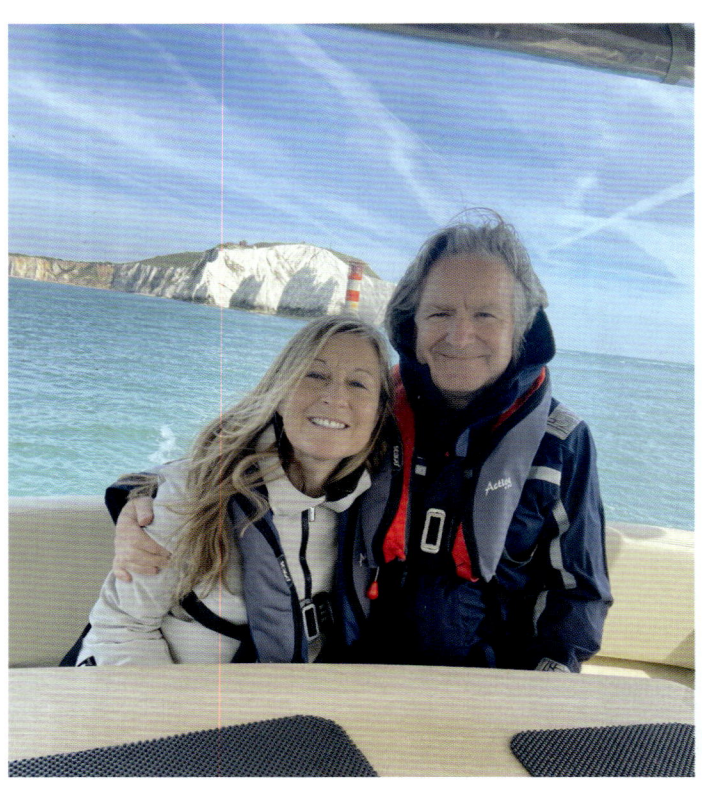

Martin and I love having new adventures together – this time on his boat at the Needles, Isle of Wight.

'You've totally zoned out of our family and our marriage,' he would say to me.

'Don't be so bloody ridiculous!' I'd yell back. 'If I've zoned out, who do you think it is who's putting the washing on twice a day or picking up those trainers all over the front room?'

But, if I'm honest, I think he was right. I just didn't seem to have the energy for any of it any more. The boys were teenagers and didn't need me as they had done when they were younger, and Martin was at work twelve hours a day, every day. That sense of not being needed as much didn't bother me, though; in fact it was a bit of a relief. In 2017, I was still working, preparing to present *Shop Smart, Save Money* on Channel 5, so I had enough to keep myself busy, though not too much. But when I was at home I just couldn't find the oomph to be the sparkly person I thought everyone expected – I'd had enough of all that.

I'm sure I wasn't easy to live with, but then Martin was hardly God's gift to marriage either. He was always at work and, when he wasn't there, he was thinking about work, setting up interviews for the following week, dealing with stories in the press that seemed to hit *This Morning* every couple of weeks. I knew it was all part of his job and perhaps more than anyone else I understood the pressures of working in TV, but that didn't make it any less annoying, so I just took a big step back and let him get on with it.

So yes, I guess we did drift apart at that point. I'm just not sure how much I realized it as I was still so caught up in grief about my parents and the hangover of the stress from work. And most days, like most people, I just got on with what had to be done – shopping, cooking, writing my column and preparing for the bits of TV work that were still coming in.

We still had good times together. Occasionally we still went out for dinner, but more often than not if Martin suggested a night out then I'd say I was too tired or couldn't face it. Maybe the following week?

The whole idea of 'date nights' that they bang on about in women's magazines makes me feel sick – as if our parents' generation ever did anything so silly as that!

We had some wonderful holidays at our little house in Italy – I loved that it was so quiet and hidden away from the world. But then we would be back to London and reality. Back to bickering over who should put the bins out and long silences over dinner.

Things weren't great, but I didn't realize quite how seriously Martin felt about it all until one evening he dropped an absolute bombshell.

'I'm moving out,' he said. 'I just think we need some time apart. And I think you need to decide whether you still want to be in this marriage.'

'Oh, for God's sake, Martin!' I yelled. 'Stop being so ridiculous. I'm just worn out. I'm tired – of everything.'

'That's what you've been saying for years,' he replied. 'Maybe this – our marriage – is what's making you so tired.'

At this point, I didn't even argue back. I didn't think he was right; I didn't think for one moment my relationship with him was what was behind me feeling so down about everything. It was something else that I had no means of controlling, but I couldn't ever seem to explain that properly.

So off he went to a hotel with his toothbrush and a small bag of clothes. I took the small size of the bag as a positive sign – clearly, he wasn't thinking of staying away a long time. Or was he? I really didn't know and that felt incredibly scary.

My husband had been the one constant in my life through everything that had happened over the past two decades and it seemed unbelievable that he might not be there in the future. I don't think I ever thought he would leave me completely. It felt much more like he was trying to shock me into behaving differently or prod us both out of the marriage slump we'd found ourselves in.

And it worked. Even though we had been distant for months and months, I missed Martin. And if I did think about what a future might be like without him, it just seemed bewildering.

A sort of nothingness.

The first week he was gone was a bit of a blur. I was angry that he'd just upped and left, but I was too proud to call and beg him to come home. By the second week, I was beginning to wonder how long he was planning on keeping this up. I knew he was ringing the boys to check we were all OK, but mainly to find out if I'd been pining for him!

'How's Dad?' I'd ask Nat and Mackenzie as casually as I could manage. 'Where's he staying? I really think he should come home now – he's made his point.'

It was only a fortnight, but it felt like he had been away for months. The thought that he might never come back started to grow in my mind. I did spend time thinking about how I'd behaved towards him, not just in the past few months, but over the years when I'd been so preoccupied with my parents and work. Not that I regretted that for a moment, but clearly it had taken its toll on our marriage.

By the third week of our separation, we had started texting each other and then we spoke on the phone.

'So are you planning on coming home then?' I asked, trying to find that fine line between appearing to care without seeming desperate.

But Martin was still playing hardball. 'I'm not coming home until we've sorted things out between us,' he said. 'We can't just slip into how things were before.'

He wanted us to meet to talk everything through, so he booked a beautiful hotel in Hampshire for one Friday evening. It was very sweet of him and I took that as a sign he wanted to get things back on track – and so did I.

Driving down, I felt nervous in a way that I hadn't for years. After three weeks, I desperately wanted my husband home. For all the arguments and the bickering and my moaning, I still loved him – I always had done. I wanted him back, I wanted myself back. I just wasn't sure whether I could do it.

That evening was difficult – but great. Without allowing things to descend into another row, Martin explained how he had been feeling.

'You've been so distant for so long,' he told me. 'I just need to know – is this going to work or not?'

'Well, I want it to work,' I said.

'And so do I,' he said. 'But things have got to change.'

And I knew he was right. I knew it – I just didn't know how to change things.

18

Menopause. It had to be the menopause.

Suddenly everything made perfect sense – why I'd been feeling so strange for so long. I spent hours reading up online about symptoms and it all seemed to tally: loss of concentration, sleeplessness, brain fog, feeling down and depressed. I had all of those things – that's what it had to be.

Around this time lots of women in the public eye like Davina McCall and Gabby Logan were discussing menopause in a way it had never been talked about before. It felt like all the pieces were falling into place – why hadn't anyone told me before how debilitating the menopause could be?

But I didn't have the hot flushes that a lot of women complain about – for me it was the sense of brain fog and a sense of anxiety that I could rarely shake off. The brain fog had become increasingly common. I'd be halfway through a sentence and then forget what I'd been planning to say. Or I'd read a story in the newspaper in the morning then be completely unable to remember what the point of it was. I started making lists all the time – shopping lists, to-do lists. If I was chatting to a friend or my agent on the phone, I would quickly write down what we had discussed in case it dropped out of my mind straight after.

The other awful feeling was the aching anxiety that seemed to be with me so much of the time. Increasingly, things I'd done for decades, like turning up to film a programme, made me feel sick with nerves. I kept pushing myself to do them as part of me was desperate to work, but the other part was terrified by the prospect of it.

Online, I found a herbal progesterone and oestrogen cream. Friends had suggested I should go to my GP and ask for HRT, but my research had shown that the types they prescribed were animal-based and, as a vegetarian, I didn't want that. Instead, I started using a plant-based cream called Organic Excellence. Each morning and evening, I'd rub in a blob at the top of my arms or stomach. Everything I read said that within a month or so I would be feeling back to my old self.

Except, after six months of daily treatment, I wasn't quite sure whether it had really kicked in yet.

Some days I'd wake up feeling fine, full of vim and vigour and ready to work, and I was convinced the cream was doing its job. But then other days I just felt so low.

For years I'd read every national newspaper each morning to know what was going on in the world in preparation for writing my *Mirror* column on a Thursday. I'd take the huge pile of papers up to the office and work my way through them with a cup of tea and my laptop to type any notes. But increasingly I found it hard to concentrate when reading, let alone find anything I thought worth taking notes about. My mind would wander off halfway down a page or I'd just lose interest and go downstairs to make another cup of tea.

By the time I got to Thursday, I was in a flat panic about what to write. Each week I'd manage to rattle something out and I'd answer the dozens of readers' letters I still received each day. But when I thought about the big news issues, the never-ending attempts by PM Theresa May to get a Brexit deal done or even the preparations for Prince Harry and Meghan Markle's spring 2018 wedding, I just couldn't summon up much enthusiasm. It felt like the ever-growing pile of unread newspapers was taunting me for my failure to do my job and that just made me feel more anxious than ever.

I wrote about the menopause a few times in my *Mirror* column – I felt it was important to share my experiences so that other women going through the same thing would feel less alone. Then in June 2018, my friend Lorraine Kelly invited me onto her daytime TV show for an interview, after I'd written again about the impact I felt the menopause was having on me. She wanted to discuss a subject that impacted so many of her viewers but for years had been almost entirely taboo.

I talked about how my mum had suffered horribly through the menopause and as a young woman I'd raised my eyebrows and thought, *Oh come on, surely it can't be as bad as all that?* But now I was finding out that for some women, including myself, it was that bad – it was absolutely horrendous.

I tried to explain what anxiety felt like, particularly when for the most part of my life I'd been entirely independent and nothing would faze me. Now the simplest thing like going to the bank to ask about my account would send me into a total panic.

I didn't talk about it on *Lorraine*, but there were mood swings too, which meant even I was finding my behaviour unpredictable, so goodness knows how hard it must have been for Martin and the boys to read. And yet, despite not wanting to be like that, I couldn't do anything about it. I felt I'd lost control over my own life, and that made me feel vulnerable and anxious – it was all a terrible vicious circle.

Throughout all this, I kept much of what I was feeling to myself. I didn't want to go on to Martin about it and besides what was the point? He couldn't do anything to help – it was just a stage of life I was going through even if it was causing chaos in his life too!

When I thought back to how Mum had suffered, I felt guilty for all those times I hadn't thought to offer more support when she locked herself away in her room, in her mid-fifties, and cried. Back then, GPs didn't know how to treat menopause – or even care about it. They were almost all men and the whole healthcare system pretty much ignored the other half of the population, particularly anything involving hormones, what they'd call 'women's business'.

Now it was happening to me. Hopefully I'd get through it soon. The menopause couldn't last for ever. Unless of course, it was something . . . else. But I wasn't going to go there.

Some people reading this story will think the similarities

between my parents' stories and my own are overwhelming. When I went on the *Lorraine* show, I was fifty-seven – about the same age my mum had been suffering from anxiety and depression. And of course I knew exactly what had come next for Mum. We had never known for certain whether her anxiety and menopause symptoms had been just that or actually early symptoms of Alzheimer's. In my mind I became more determined that for Mum, they had been entirely separate things. Would you have chosen to think differently? Remember, this is a terminal illness we are considering. I refused to let my mind see the patterns that were emerging.

19

Martin

You'll be looking at me too, won't you?

Most likely you're saying to yourself, 'Surely the similarities between Fiona's mother's condition and her own were too striking? Surely, on some level, she must have feared something more serious was also happening to her?' And you'll be asking why on earth I didn't raise the alarm sooner as my wife went through that depression and then those symptoms of menopause.

You'll be wondering why as bright, educated people we didn't think this might be the beginning – the start of Alzheimer's stealth attack on Fiona's mind.

I honestly don't know. All I can say is at the time I really didn't think so.

I guess this book, as with all autobiographies, shines a light on the key moments of Fiona's life. And a lot of those were times of trauma and sadness. But there were many, many more moments when we were just a fairly ordinary family doing the things ordinary families do – watching the football with the boys on a Saturday afternoon, spinning around the supermarket, stocking up on washing powder and teabags, visiting relatives, celebrating birthdays, going on holiday, watching TV. We were just getting on with life and enjoying it as we could, rather than having a laser focus on the things that weren't quite right. It's only looking back that the patterns become visible – I suppose that's the perspective of distance.

As Fiona has explained, we had been struggling in our marriage for a while – probably from about 2015. Fiona became very distant with me and she even seemed detached with the children. I was worried about the future of our relationship – I felt she was critical of everything we did and she was also withdrawn and silent. She'd become really moody, even though Fiona had never been a moody person before. She'd always been totally upfront about how she felt and didn't sulk about things, but now there seemed a hidden anger towards us all. It was as if she resented us and the fact that she had felt so low for so long.

For years we avoided bringing tensions in the house to a head, probably because I always acquiesced to her and agreed with whatever she said, so things didn't really fester much. But by then I'd probably had enough of saying 'yes' to everything. And even my saying 'yes' wasn't enough to improve her mood. Nothing I could say seemed to help.

And I guess like in any relationship, the whole thing spirals. Because I felt she was being moody and critical of everything I said and did, I shut down too. We were barely talking and while we were still in the same house we were living quite separate lives.

If we were both at home in the evenings, there would be long silences. After years of being able to chat about anything and everything, we'd run out of things to talk about. The long silences can't have been enjoyable for her either, but that was where we had got to. I didn't think for one moment that it was the menopause or, perish the thought, Alzheimer's. I just thought we had hit the wall that so many marriages do as the kids get older – ours were now well into their teens – and maybe as a couple we had just run our course. And because I felt Fiona was being so withdrawn and disinterested in me and the boys, I wasn't devastated by that thought.

I think Fiona knew she was being difficult but was struggling to find some meaning for the way she was feeling and perhaps wanted some relief or escape from that. It was then that I dropped my bombshell.

'This can't go on, Fiona,' I said, one evening. 'It's making us all miserable. I'm going to move out for a couple of weeks – I'll find a hotel. Maybe you can use the time to work out what you really want and then we can see if there's anything left of this marriage.'

Like Fiona says, it was a very difficult few weeks. We spoke on the phone and she asked me to return, but I was determined not to run straight back or for things to simply revert to the way they had been before. I needed her to look at the way she had been behaving towards all of us, but most of all I was hoping this might shock her out of the awful slump she had been in for so long. And I think it worked – a bit. She had a kind of reset while I was away.

That evening when we had our meeting in the hotel in Hampshire was great. We were laughing and chatting as if the previous ten years had never happened. And it was amazing. I knew how much I loved Fiona – I'd always loved her and I didn't want our family and home to be torn apart.

It was clear that we both wanted the marriage to continue and Fiona accepted she had been distant for a long time, but there was no discussion as to what lay behind the distance.

After I came home, things were better. Clearly my moving out had given Fiona a bit of a jolt and for a while she was more engaged in what the rest of us were doing. She was more chatty and easier to be with, but deep down I knew there was still this underlying thing. I knew something wasn't right.

Gradually our lives slipped back into the same sad pattern. I reverted to simply parking any concerns at the back of my mind. It's incredible in day-to-day life how you can just not tackle the things you don't want to deal with.

The knowledge that me and our family were no longer able to make Fiona happy was so painful that I buried it deep down, somewhere I didn't have to process it.

The media was full of previously high-functioning women talking about how debilitating they'd found the menopause. How it had totally changed their personality. And big debates were going on about whether women should be able to take time off work with menopause symptoms.

Everything I read and watched on TV pointed firmly to the fact Fiona was right and it must be the menopause causing her symptoms. That was when she started to struggle. And if it was menopause then logically the symptoms would pass and she would be back to her old self. Or at least she would feel better.

In hindsight, was it that 'confirmation bias' thing – where you twist everything you learn to fit with what you want to believe? Maybe. Maybe . . .

And of course the alternative – that this was the beginnings of Alzheimer's – was too awful to consider, so it was not in my thinking.

During the writing of this book, I remembered a moment that might be significant. It was around this time, 2018, that Fiona became obsessed with the idea that we should clean out the loft.

'What on earth do you want to do that for?' I asked. 'It'll take ages – there's stuff up there that has been in boxes since we moved in.'

'That's exactly the reason,' she replied. 'I don't want to have to leave all that for the boys to do if we're dead and buried – we should sort it out so they don't have to.'

'But that will be years and years away – we can worry about that at some point in the future,' I told her.

But she was insistent.

'No, I want to do it now,' she said.

Did she know Alzheimer's had come for her but she couldn't consciously face that? I guess she did. She has even said so in press interviews and on television, but at home it was left unspoken. Maybe that was because we still had relatively young sons and we wouldn't want them hearing such a conversation, but it was also just too awful.

If we didn't discuss it, maybe it wasn't a real possibility.

And there were still times when she was able to lift herself and we'd have fun together on holiday in Italy or if we were out for dinner. I don't want you to think it was wall-to-wall doom and gloom. Yes, it was tough, but there were good times too and those were the moments we both focused on. And we hoped the bad moments would pass with the menopause.

Now I think someone in the early stages of Alzheimer's is so desperate for this not to be happening to them that they will fixate on any alternative – and that is perfectly understandable. Because there is no cure. At least, there is currently no cure – and everyone knows that. So obviously Fiona or anyone in this situation would hope against hope that it is something else and self-diagnose the problem rather than see a doctor.

The fear would be that a GP would tell you something you desperately do not want to hear.

20

Fiona

'I'm going to Vietnam,' I told Martin one evening over dinner in October 2019.

'Where?' he said, in that tetchy tone I had become used to.

'Vietnam,' I snapped back. 'As you clearly heard me say the first time. I've booked the tickets, I'm going next week.'

'And you didn't think to mention this sooner?' he replied. 'Or ask if I might fancy coming along? And I suppose you've not thought of telling Nat or Mackenzie either?'

He was right. I hadn't thought about whether he might want to come or told the boys yet. But I wasn't being secretive – I hadn't revealed my travel plans sooner because I hadn't known I was going myself until that morning. It all just spilled out of a conversation on the phone to my old friend Neal Harrison, who by then had given up television work and was living a life of leisure on the Indonesian island of Bali.

Although he had moved far away for a quieter life among the palm trees and white sand beaches, we had always kept in touch by phone and email. Months might go by and we wouldn't talk, but then one of us would call and we could spend a couple of hours chatting and laughing on the phone.

We had been talking that morning when Neal told me he was planning a trip over to Vietnam for a few beaches, a bit of sightseeing and some great food. With the grey London sky drilling down on me and the thought of another long winter ahead, I'd spoken before I'd even thought: 'I'll come. I could do with a holiday, get away from everything here.'

Within hours my flights were booked. Neal looked after everything else – booking hotels, sorting transport. It was just like the old days when we'd worked together! But first I had to break it to Martin that I was going. And as you can see, it hadn't gone well, although once I'd told him there was no big row. Just a shrug of the shoulders as he walked into the other room, scrolling through his phone.

He didn't have to say what he was thinking because I already knew: *Whatever, do what you want. You always do.* And was that fair? Well, obviously I could never admit it, but there was perhaps some truth in it. I did do what I wanted to do – but then why on earth shouldn't I? I'd spent years and years of my life putting on a smiley face at work every morning while looking after the boys and my parents. Why shouldn't I just have a little bit of fun? I was also hoping that possibly this trip might be the lift I needed to pull me out of the sense of blankness that still hadn't left me over the past year. Well, it wasn't just one year. If I thought it through, it had been going on for years now.

It was my new normal.

It is hard to describe the general sense of flatness in anything and everything that I did. There wasn't one overnight descent into confusion or darkness, it was more like a never-ending trudge down a tunnel, each step taking me further from the light. Did I still believe that 'light at the end of the tunnel' stuff? Not sure I did, to be honest.

I was still trying to write my weekly *Mirror* column, but some days my mind was so befuddled that I couldn't think of a single fresh opinion. And because I'd turned down so much TV work, the calls had dried up. It meant I was cooped up at home a lot of the time so not in a great mood when Martin got in from work. It was all right for him – he was going out every day, meeting interesting people, making big decisions about the news while I was stuck at home staring out of the window. But however much I wanted to summon up the energy to get up and out of the house, it all felt a struggle.

I guess that was a big reason relations between me and Martin hadn't been that great. I was snappy with him and the boys. It felt like there were constantly bags and coats abandoned in the front room or damp towels on the bathroom floor – and I'd be the one picking them up. They seemed to be always needing food too! Martin would want some big steak, which he'd be cooking, oozing with blood and making me feel sick. As a vegetarian, the sight of raw meat has never become manageable. Sometimes it felt like everything my family did irritated me – I was just desperate for some peace and quiet. Often I'd go and sit in another room just to be on my own.

There were no blazing rows between me and Martin – we

were just talking less and less. Sometimes he'd get frustrated and say: 'Why do you have to criticize everything I do?' Other times he'd really try to get through to me and ask if I fancied going out for dinner, but I couldn't face the hassle of getting ready and having to chat all evening so I'd just shrug.

'You've got no interest in me, the boys or anything,' he told me. 'You're being utterly selfish.'

Years ago, I'd have been at him like a rattlesnake for saying something like that, but now I really couldn't be bothered. It was all just too exhausting and what was the point in rowing anyway? So I really did think that the trip to Vietnam would be good for me – and Martin. A bit of a break from each other.

Maybe it could even be the thing to bring me out of my slump. When Martin had left for a few weeks it had kickstarted things for a while and maybe this would do the same. A bit of time away to consider how I felt if maybe, just maybe, something very bad was starting to happen to me.

In October 2019, I flew into Hanoi in north Vietnam and met Neal straight away. It was wonderful to see him again. He had sorted the entire itinerary for us in advance and there were guides to meet us in every town and city we were staying in.

In Hanoi, our guide spotted and introduced us to Phan Thi Kim Phuc, who was famously the 'napalm girl' in the iconic Pulitzer Prize-winning photo taken on 8 June 1972, which showed her aged nine, running down a road naked after having been terribly burned in a napalm attack. The 'Terror of War' image came to symbolize the horror of the Vietnam War, but she had survived her injuries and gone on to campaign for child victims of conflict.

Phan was such a friendly, warm woman and we felt privileged to have met her. That incredible chance encounter, which was so fascinating, reminded me of all the chance encounters we'd had with well-known folk during our LA years.

Afterwards we took a seaplane over Halong Bay and sailed through the islands before flying down to Hoi An. We then had a bit of time relaxing on white sand beaches on the island of Con Dao, looking out at the perfect turquoise sea. Finally, we went to Saigon, where we had a trip down the Mekong river and explored the infamous Vietcong tunnels.

There were so many new experiences that I did feel revitalized by the trip and it was nice to have time to talk to Neal about how I'd really been feeling too. I was able to share with him some of my deepest, darkest fears. What if this wasn't actually stress or menopause? What if it was something much more serious?

We talked quite a bit about how Alzheimer's has a terrible way of eating away at people. Neal's mum had suffered from it, so he knew how awful it can be. I even mentioned the new drugs that were being developed and how I could try taking Lecanemab, which is known to slow Alzheimer's in its early stages, if that was what I really did have. With Neal, I could also share the fears I had about how people would judge me if I were to have Alzheimer's – I had absolutely no desire for something so personal to become public property.

Even on that magical trip, there were a couple of times when the sense of confusion came over me. Once we were in a hotel and I spent an hour looking at my suitcase, wondering what I had forgotten to put in it. I knew the item was missing, but I couldn't think what it was – it was all so strange. And other times I just felt anxious, even when I was surrounded by the most dazzling scenery and my closest friend. Those moments soon passed, though, and most of the time I felt fine – Neal and I laughed and chatted from morning until night.

Most of the time, I felt at peace.

21

Martin

—————

Maybe I should step in here and explain how things appeared to me at home when Fiona announced her trip to Vietnam in 2019. As she has explained, I was more than a bit shocked. It was just entirely out of the blue without any thought as to how the boys and I might feel about it – and it was also pretty much out of character. While this was the sort of thing she might have done without blinking an eye ten years earlier, for the past couple of years it had been an effort to get her to go anywhere.

The sad reality by then, though, was that it came as a bit of a relief for me and the boys because Fiona hadn't been pleasant to be around for a while. The idea that she would be gone for a fortnight seemed like a respite. It's hard to say that because it sounds terrible and now I understand the reason she had been so difficult to live with was because she may already have been suffering from the disease that would take her away from us for ever. But the cold reality of this illness is that it changes people's behaviour slowly over such a long period that those living around them don't have one blinding moment of realization that their partner is ill, they just know they have changed.

Of course, maybe I should have understood her sudden decision to up and go to Vietnam was another indication that things were not all they should be, but at the time it just felt like another thread being pulled in our fraying marriage. And it's not like Fiona and I had always been joined at the hip the way some couples are. We'd both remained pretty independent the whole time we were together, in a healthy way. I'd never been jealous or tried to control anything Fiona wanted to do and I knew there was nothing more than friendship between her and Neal, so that wasn't the issue — it was the way she announced it.

Normally, Fiona would have asked me what I thought about the trip or she would certainly have explained what she was planning on doing, but that time it was just, 'right, I'm upping sticks and going'. I hoped that going to see an old friend and having an adventure far from home might shake things up for her. She was heading towards her sixties and it's not just men who have midlife crises, women do too. Maybe she thought that's what it was and she just needed to go and reconnect with herself as well as her old friend and have a good time away from her family. Maybe she was thinking, *I've given them the best years of my life. I've worked hard, brought up two kids and looked after a husband, and now it's my time to do what I want — because I'm not happy where I am.*

And that was entirely right and understandable.

Looking back, I can see how she might have believed the

trip would help her find herself again because she'd been so lost. Or perhaps she saw something coming down the line and thought she had to do something thrilling because she might not have much time left. I don't know if that would have been a conscious or subconscious feeling – or maybe it wasn't there at all. I don't know . . . Like so much, I just don't know. And at that time the pair of us weren't in a place where we could discuss what she was really feeling. But when Fiona set off on that trip I did wonder what would be left of our marriage by the time she returned.

Fiona and Neal had an amazing time. They saw some great things, had fun and loved being together, so it was a proper break for her, but I think it also made her miss me and the boys too, so she was glad to get home. And, at first, when she got back, she was in far better spirits and less withdrawn. It felt like some time away had worked. But gradually, once again, we fell back into the same routines. Some days she would barely speak to me or the boys at all. She had no interest in doing anything or going anywhere and it was grinding us all down. I wasn't aware that Fiona had broached the idea that she might have Alzheimer's with Neal. As far as I was concerned, we both remained convinced that the problem was the menopause – I certainly hoped that was all it was – and so we continued plodding along.

22

Fiona

In February 2020, Covid hit. What started as concerns about a few people arriving in Britain who might have been infected evolved very quickly into terror about a pandemic killing thousands. The world was turned upside down.

Poor Nat had just been accepted into the army at that point. He had turned into such a big, strong man with an equally big heart and he'd dreamed of going into the army for years. He loved the idea of travelling and doing something of value for his country. I just dreaded the thought of him being far from home or getting hurt or even killed. But it was his dream and neither Martin nor I were going to stand in the way of it.

But just as Nat was about to start his training that spring, the national lockdown hit, so instead of an exciting future with new mates running around on manouevres, he was incarcerated at home with the rest of the family. But in those first sunny days of the lockdown, we had good times together. We would sit and eat as a family some evenings, which we hadn't done for years. And we would go for walks on the Common and chat.

It was a reminder of when the boys were younger and all our lives revolved around the home that bit more.

But only a few weeks into the pandemic, I was struck down with a terrible stomach ache and that dry cough. Yep, I'd caught Covid. Goodness knows where I'd caught it from as I had barely been out. It totally koshed me over the head and I felt dreadful. I went to bed and barely had the energy to get up for a glass of water.

At first I was utterly shattered. I slept for days on end, sweating and coughing. It was as if a witch had shoved her twiggy broom up into my alimentary canal and into my throat, left it there and then intermittently twisted it. I had a horrible pain in my guts and my entire body ached. My appetite went completely. Martin tried to keep his distance from me as he didn't want to catch it – but he was great and kept popping up to the bedroom with jugs of water and cups of tea. I felt so rotten and there was a point when I thought it would never end.

I felt rough for three weeks, listless and knocked out. But when I watched the news and saw how horrendously some people were suffering, I was grateful it hadn't been worse. Even when the worst of Covid had passed, I still felt shattered. At least with the national lockdown continuing I didn't even have to make excuses for not wanting to go out – because no one was allowed to!

It was a terrible time for those with preexisting health conditions and, night after night, we would see on our television the plight of people in care homes, who had effectively been abandoned by those in power. When it emerged later that patients with Covid had been allowed to go back into care homes, where they spread the disease to otherwise healthy residents, it made my blood boil. It seemed as if elderly people – particularly those with dementia – were at the bottom of everyone's lists, as if they were dispensable.

Hundreds of them died when they could have been saved. And the idea that they spent their last days alone, without loved ones by their side because of the restrictions on entering care homes, was heartbreaking.

The terrible realities of the pandemic were everywhere. Martin and I were devastated when our friend Derek Draper, the political lobbyist, was taken into hospital in March of that year after catching the virus. Derek was married to my good friend and fellow broadcaster Kate Garraway, with whom I had worked at *GMTV*. She presented on the days when I didn't, so we were constantly chatting about stories and all the behind-the-scenes gossip. Even after I left in 2008, we kept in touch, and sometimes Kate, Derek, Martin and I would go out together – they were great fun.

For someone we knew well to be in hospital with this awful illness hammered home just how bad it was. I kept in touch with Kate as Derek's condition quickly deteriorated and he was placed on a ventilator and put into an induced coma to give his body the best chance of survival. Poor Kate was sick with worry and she had two young children to look after too – it was horrendous for them all.

Around this time the Alzheimer's Society, for whom I had

regularly done work since my parents were ill, asked if I would do a public appeal for fundraising. They were desperate for cash because so much of their fundraising had stopped and shops closed due to the pandemic. Meanwhile the demand for their services was going through the roof as sufferers and their families felt isolated with nowhere else to turn.

Glad to help in some small way, I recorded a short appeal asking people to donate to the charity, explaining how vital any contribution would be to help those suffering with the illness during the pandemic. I'd always tried to support the Alzheimer's Society because of the incredible work they do in supporting those with the illness and carrying out leading research into its causes and treatment – little did I know then how desperate I would soon be for a breakthrough in that research.

In the summer of 2020, the Covid restrictions were eased and life for many people returned to something approaching normal. We were allowed to go to pubs and restaurants again, visit family and even go on holiday. For our friends Kate and Derek, however, the nightmare continued. Derek remained in intensive care. It was a year later when he was finally allowed home, but by then that awful illness had ravaged his body, leaving him weak and exhausted. Tragically, Derek died in January 2024. Kate had done a superhuman job looking after him and their children.

Anything I was going through seemed trivial in comparison, yet gradually, very gradually, so gradually in fact that it was impossible to tell, the anxiety and brain fog were getting worse. I started to think I must be suffering from Long Covid.

From the summer of 2020, there was a lot in the news about Long Covid. Thousands of people who had suffered Covid were reporting similar symptoms – terrible exhaustion, difficulty sleeping, memory loss and breathlessness. It was thought as many as 7 per cent of all those who caught Covid could be impacted. And it tallied exactly with how I was feeling. I had the most terrible lethargy and couldn't be bothered to do anything. But, even though I was constantly shattered, my sleep was poor and I could toss and turn for hours at night. It was so soon after Covid that there had been hardly any research into the condition. Doctors had no idea if it would pass or whether it could become a chronic condition.

By June, I was so concerned about how I was feeling that I wrote my *Mirror* column all about it. They headlined the article: 'Not alone in battling cruel Covid hangover'. So you can see exactly how I was feeling then, this is what I wrote:

Recently, I seem to have been replaced by a person I'm not familiar with. I don't like this jittery, over-the-top anxious woman. Nor the panicky cipher who can't see things for looking.

Nor the one who goes food shopping and totally forgets what she needs to buy, then panics and leaves. Nor the tearful, insecure mum, whose personality change has prompted frequent knowing looks between her two sons.

Or the one who last week pulled out of two work engagements because she couldn't stand the thought of the panic that attempting to carry them out would bring on.

Sadly, I am far from alone in experiencing this horrible Covid hangover. I'm just one of an army of people still battling the ghastly thing. I think about my friend Derek Draper – still on a ventilator – each and every day.

I know (hope?) my symptoms will fade with time. I am desperate for them to hop on the bus to viral extinction.

In the meantime, I'm having weekly hypnotherapy sessions and using a high-concentration CBD oil to calm my frazzled nerves.

Just hoping they'll bring me back to who I was again. And very much wishing the same for others, who've had the misfortune to be touched by this cruel, vile virus.

The symptoms seemed to stay with me for the remainder of 2020. Did I really think I was suffering Long Covid or was I using that as another excuse to the world for why my behaviour had changed? Or was I using that as an excuse to *myself*? Now I struggle to know. Maybe it was a combination of all those things.

Like I said in my column, I was now going for weekly hypnotherapy sessions with a therapist near my home. He would try to find a way to help me manage my anxiety – but it didn't work.

CBD (cannabidiol) oil is extracted from hemp plants (*Cannabis sativa*) and there is a lot of research that shows it can help people suffering with mood disorders and can help reduce symptoms of depression, anxiety and even psychosis. I did feel that the CBD oil helped, but still I wasn't my old self.

The only work I felt able to even consider was writing my *Mirror* column, and that was becoming increasingly difficult. I'd sit down at my desk, open my laptop and prepare to write, then find I couldn't settle my thoughts on any subject to discuss. And, when I did make myself write something, anything, the words wouldn't flow like they used to do.

More than once, I rang in saying I felt too poorly to be able to write. The features editor, Clare Fitzsimons, was incredibly understanding. Some weeks she would even help me put together what I wanted to say when I was struggling to find the words to express it. My contract stated I was supposed to write a column every week, but I was wondering how much longer I could keep it up. One week I wrote a column almost identical to the one from the previous week, which couldn't be published. I was mortified, but Clare was so lovely. And, because lots of people knew someone struggling with Long Covid at that time, I think it was genuinely accepted that this was what was causing me so much difficulty.

By November the following year, though, I needed a total break from everything. I asked for a couple of months off work while I tried to sort myself out. Thankfully, I'd worked for them for so long that they agreed.

'I'll be back in the New Year, though, I promise.'

We had a good Christmas with the boys. I loved the idea of being able to close the front door and our family being all together. It felt so much less stressful than the demands of the outside world. Martin looked after all the cooking so there really was nothing for me to worry about, but of course the anxiety and worry remained. As did the tears. I just felt so vulnerable.

By the New Year, I was a little better. Or at least I managed to convince myself I was feeling better. I returned to writing the column – and thought I owed my readers a proper explanation of what had been going on. I didn't want them thinking I'd been swanning around on some beach in the Caribbean over New Year when really, I'd been at home trying to summon up the courage to step out the front door.

I told them how it felt I'd cried a thousand rivers over the past few weeks even though I knew I had nothing to be sad about. I knew there were women and children dying in war zones all over the world and then here was me with a happy, healthy family and all I could do was cry.

I also shared with them the thing that was lurking beneath: 'I've been fearing for my sanity.' But despite that, in the same breath, I kept blaming the menopause too. Perhaps it was easier to talk about the menopause and to campaign for better understanding of the conditions and treatments for women than to consider what else might be happening.

'I don't know what I'm talking about half the time,' I told my *Mirror* readers. I went on:

And it's this constant fear I'm living with. God, it's horrible. I haven't worked for the first time in my life, I can't do television work because I'm so anxious and just scared of everything and I'm not that kind of person at all. I have the intent to do everything I used to do, but then your body, your brain, doesn't let you.

The fear takes over. I hope to God this isn't the end of my career.

The thought that I might never work again loomed large at that time. Work was still how I defined myself, so if I wasn't able to work, what actually was I? But, at the same time, I felt I wasn't able to function as a mother either.

Mackenzie was still living with us, but Nat had finally been able to start his army training and was absolutely loving it. Because he was still in the early stages of it all, he was allowed home every weekend. I loved seeing him walk through the door on a Friday evening, strong and full of stories about what he'd been up to all week, but from about Thursday morning I would be panicking about what on earth I was going to cook for his dinner when he got home.

'What shall I make?' I'd say to Martin. 'I just can't decide. I could do a lasagna, but maybe he won't fancy that. Or a casserole? But I'm not sure I'll be able to make it properly. It won't be right or he might not like it.'

What should have been a simple thing became a massive issue.

'Don't worry about it,' Martin would say. 'I'll cook or we can have a takeaway. It's not a big deal.'

But it was a big deal for me – it was a massive deal. And the thought I couldn't knock up a quick casserole for my eldest son just made me feel hopeless.

Around then, I also lost my confidence around driving. I'd been driving since I passed my test at seventeen. For years I'd nipped round London in my little Mini and then I did those epic trips back and forth to Wales with two little kids in the back. But now just the thought of driving through the streets near our home made my palms sweat and I felt sick. The roads were all so busy – and what if I forgot which pedal to press or which street to go down?

Even popping to the shops, which I had done a million times before, became terrifying. One day I was standing in the aisle in Sainsbury's and I was overcome with anxiety. I could feel my heart racing and I thought I was going to pass out – I just couldn't cope with being there. I abandoned my shopping trolley in the middle of the aisle, rushed out and sat in the car until I calmed down. Although I tried to summon the strength to go back in and finish the shop, I couldn't do it – I couldn't go back into my local Sainsbury's. I just drove home and stayed indoors for the rest of the day. I was utterly unable to explain what specifically had made me so anxious: it was just there.

The anxiety attacks became more frequent until they were almost hourly. Then that sense of anxiety was with me, to some degree, all the time. Martin could see how distressing I was finding things. I think he might have been keen for me to go to see a doctor who could assess me properly, but he also knew I hated the idea of being poked and peered at by a bunch of physicians in white coats.

During 2021, Dr Louise Newson had been appearing frequently on Martin's show, *This Morning*. Dr Newson had at that point become known as the UK's leading expert on menopause. She was leading research into the conditions, its symptoms and treatments; she was also hosting a podcast and launched an app called Balance. Finally, it felt as if menopause was being treated seriously as an issue. There were dozens of newspaper articles and television programmes focused on it.

When Dr Newson made one of her first appearances on *This Morning* in May 2021, the show was contacted by more than 7,000 women who were all concerned about the menopause. It seemed to be this awful secret epidemic that had been going on for years and destroying the lives of so many women like me.

Martin said that if the way I was feeling was down to menopause then Dr Newson was the person to diagnose it.

'So, if I make an appointment, will you go and see Dr Newson?' he asked me.

My cynicism about doctors remained and I was still uncertain. But I was also becoming desperate for some help from someone. I agreed to go along for blood tests to check my hormone levels and work out what the best course of treatment could be. I felt like I'd become half a person – I longed to regain the half that I'd lost.

23

Martin

———

By the start of 2022, I was pinning a lot of hope on Dr Louise Newson. The previous twelve months had been incredibly difficult. It felt Fiona was slipping further and further away from me, Nat and Mackenzie.

If I suggested going out for dinner or going away for a weekend, Fiona would say: 'No, I don't want to do it, I'll just stay here.' But even if she stayed indoors, she wasn't doing anything specific. She would tidy up – she has always been quite fastidious. Or she might make some lunch or occasionally see her friend Amanda, who'd had sons at school with our boys, but overall, she did very little. For a long while we didn't do much as a couple or a family.

People talk about 'crippling anxiety' and that is exactly what Fiona had. Some days she couldn't do anything because she was so anxious about the world, overwhelmed and tearful. She was physically crippled by it.

With Fiona struggling so much, I thought she really needed to see a menopause specialist. I mentioned it a few times, but she was very reluctant about seeing any proper doctors. She hoped some of the alternative cures, such as CBD oil and hypnotherapy, would help, but even she was beginning to realize it might be time to go down a more conventional route.

It was then that I suggested going to see Dr Newson. Fiona didn't even have the energy to make the appointment herself, so I organized it all and took her along to the first session. By then, I guess, I had growing concerns that what was happening was something more than menopause, but I hated the thought of that so I pinned my hopes on the alternatives.

Dr Newson was lovely. She had a long chat with Fiona and took blood tests. She also put her on a course of hormone replacement therapy. If it was the menopause then within a couple of months the brain fog and anxiety symptoms should have started to ease.

Fiona had always been nervous of taking HRT as she was convinced it was what had caused her mum's breast cancer. Back in the 1990s and early 2000s, there had been a lot of media reports that there might be a link between the two, but this has since been discredited. And, regardless of any previous concerns, she was so desperate to get better that she was prepared to take the synthetic HRT – a mixture of oestrogen, progesterone and testosterone.

We waited a couple of months to see if there was any discernible change in her condition. I hoped against hope that the brain fog would ease, but there were no obvious signs that it was. It was around this time that I really started to worry, particularly about the memory issues. Fiona would go upstairs and then come down again a few minutes later, looking upset and confused.

I'd say, 'Why did you go upstairs?', but she couldn't remember. That kind of thing was becoming more frequent and I had a horrible sick feeling about what the reality might be. And probably even more worrying than the memory loss was the anxiety – that was the big thing. Fiona wasn't suffering full-on hysterical attacks where she couldn't function, but she would have times when she was very panicky and had a growing general anxiety.

If we were invited anywhere, she wouldn't want to go. She would say: 'I can't explain why but I just don't want to be there. I don't know what to say, I don't look right, the food won't be right.' She would make up any excuse and it was clearly so upsetting for her that I wasn't going to force her to do anything that made her feel that anxious.

I was thinking more and more often, *This is not right, this is not just depression or the menopause.* Fiona's condition was becoming 'something', but because we all know how awful that 'something' could be – a terminal disease with no escape route – it was truly terrifying to think about.

The boys just thought it was 'Mum being Mum', because she hadn't been herself for a couple of years and I suppose we had all grown a bit used to the way she was being, so it wasn't like there was one defining moment that stood out. It was a gradual decline.

At that point, I reckon Fiona didn't want to think about what was happening and was happy for me to take over sorting appointments or getting her prescriptions. I would often help apply her HRT cream to her arms and buy healthy food to make nutritious dinners – anything I could think of to get her better.

In hindsight, maybe Fiona was a few steps ahead of me in understanding what was happening to her, but she couldn't – or wouldn't – let on about what that was. I'm really not sure. But then no one can be sure. The whole point of this horrible disease, because it's happening in an individual's mind, is that no one else can really understand how it is manifesting itself to them – we can't understand the different twists and turns their mind takes as the disease takes over. The speed at which it advances is different for everyone and the symptoms can be very different. I guess that's why we are generally so bad as a society at spotting it. When someone feels a lump in their body, they instinctively know it could be cancer. Alzheimer's is so much more nuanced to detect.

When Fiona's condition failed to improve after a few months of the HRT treatment, I contacted Dr Newson again.

'The cream doesn't seem to be helping,' I explained. 'What do you think we should do next?'

The doctor read through Fiona's notes again and then said the words I'd been hoping for so long never to hear: 'Look, I think this may be something more than menopause and Fiona needs to be properly assessed.' She suggested a contact of hers, regarded as a brilliant neurologist at University College Hospital London, would be an ideal person to meet Fiona.

It felt like we were stepping closer to the brutal reality awaiting us.

24

Fiona

Diagnosis

I don't really recall much of my visits to see the menopause specialist, Dr Louise Newson, but Martin sat in on all the appointments with me at my request.

As Martin explained, she prescribed me an HRT cream, which he helped to rub into my arms each day when I couldn't be bothered or had just forgotten. And I think that helped a bit, maybe, but the terrible sense of being anxious all the time just wouldn't go away. And I kept forgetting things. My head felt full of wool I couldn't untangle. I'd start making a cup of coffee then wander off and forget what I was doing. And I was forever leaving the house without my door key or my phone. That was if I did go out for a coffee with my friend Amanda or for a brisk walk. Thankfully, Mackenzie was still living at home while applying for jobs, so was always around to let me in when I'd lost my keys again.

When Louise Newson suggested to Martin that I should go to the National Hospital for Neurology and Neurosurgery, which is part of the University College London Hospitals NHS Foundation Trust (UCLH), for more tests, I wasn't thrilled about the idea but I agreed anyway. I knew exactly what they were looking for and I guess I was becoming more convinced that they would find it. But I kept on hoping against hope that it might still be something else – I badly needed someone to make me feel better.

For my first hospital appointment, the consultant, Professor Jonathan Rohrer, gave me a series of tests. He started with questions like, 'Can you tell me what 86 minus 7 is?', and then it would be 79 minus 7, then 72 minus 7 – all the way down. It was more maths than I'd done since primary school! Then the doctor pointed to the clock and asked me the time. I'd been telling the time since I was five years old, so it all felt a bit humiliating and silly. That said, I'm not sure if it was the stress of the situation but it also felt quite difficult. Finally, they produced a large piece of paper and some pens and I had to draw two rectangles. Then I had to repeat the process, but this time the rectangles had to intersect. I was so nervous and felt sick with anxiety at being so scrutinized, but I managed it all OK, I think.

Later, Martin told me that people with Alzheimer's really struggle to make the rectangles intersect – it's something to do with how the brain works that makes it particularly difficult. I felt quite chuffed I'd managed it then. Surely if my rectangles were OK, my brain must be OK too?

After the tests, I had an MRI. If you've never had a magnetic resonance imaging scan, I can't really recommend it. First of

all, you have to lie down on a cross between a bed and a supermarket conveyor belt. Everyone else leaves the room and then
the belt starts moving and you go into a little dome that makes
a drumming noise and scans you. It's a bit like those sunbeds
everyone loved back in the eighties – but without the fluores-
cent lights!

It was an exhausting day and I was glad to get home. All we
could do now was wait for the results – more waiting.

A couple of weeks later, I had an appointment back at the
hospital for the results. I felt physically sick as we sat down
facing my consultant.

'I'm really sorry,' he said, as my stomach sank deeper, 'but the
results were inconclusive.'

I felt a surge of relief. 'Inconclusive' – that meant I couldn't
have Alzheimer's otherwise they'd have spotted it there and
then, surely? But it wasn't quite so straightforward. The doctor
was still speaking . . . 'So I'm afraid we will have to get you back
in again, this time for a lumbar puncture.'

'What's that?' I asked.

I'd heard of the procedure before, but I thought it was something to do with how people had an epidural administered if
they were in terrible pain having a baby – I didn't think it could
have anything to do with the brain.

'Well, what we do is inject into your spinal column and take
a sample of spinal fluid. Your brain and spine are all connected
so once we have that fluid, we send it off for analysis and this
will be the definitive test for whether you have Alzheimer's
or not.'

'OK,' I replied.

There was no option but to keep on trying to find out what was happening to me and then hopefully, maybe, depending on what they found, there might be some kind of cure.

I was back at the hospital a few weeks later for the lumbar puncture appointment. This time I had to lie on my side on a bed while they injected me to take the fluid sample. It was incredibly painful – horrendous. But as the doctor extracted the fluid they needed to test, I heard him saying: 'Oh, that's good, clear fluid.'

I was elated. Surely that meant I was going to be OK? That had to be a positive sign. If I was there for them to test my spinal fluid and it was coming out 'good' and 'clear', I assumed I must be OK. Maybe the worst of my fears wouldn't be real-ized after all. You might think I was kidding myself, but I truly believed there must be an alternative cause for the way I'd been feeling.

I went home with a spring in my step and, for the next few weeks, I felt so much better. Martin and I nipped off for a fortnight in Italy. I felt twenty years younger. The sense of dread and anxiety had been lifted. I could even have a laugh over a couple of glasses of wine in the evenings.

During the day, we would take drives to nearby towns, wander around the shops and cool off in cafes. Or we would sit in the shade and relax. I felt so peaceful. Martin and I were getting on well – the entire holiday was a dream.

Back home, I'd barely unpacked the suitcase and got the

washing on before we were due at the hospital again for the results of the tests. It was a sunny morning in May 2022 when we drove once more to the National Hospital for Neurology and Neurosurgery, near Russell Square. It is a hugely impressive place – part of UCLH and home to some of Britain's leading research into the nervous system and brain. As we waited in the reception area, doctors in white coats were swishing up and down the corridor and it all seemed so calm and methodical. I was desperately anxious and nervous and I kept fidgeting in my chair while everything around me appeared so still and controlled. Maybe that feeling of order was why I couldn't quite believe that my life was about to be knocked entirely off its moorings.

After a short while, Martin and I were called into the office of my consultant. He smiled as we walked in and invited us to sit down. I was trying to read anything I could into his face. He looked very serious, but then he always did. Still my hoping against hope went on.

Martin and I sat next to each other across the desk from the consultant. We made some small talk about the weather as I scanned the desk for any stray reports or letters that might give me a glimpse as to what was coming my way.

'Yes, so your results are back,' he said slowly. 'And yes, I'm afraid to tell you that you do have early-onset Alzheimer's disease.'

Martin and I stared at him. Neither of us said a word. Neither of us moved a muscle. The consultant's words hung in the air like some kind of nuclear dust. We sat rigid, locked in suspended animation between everything our lives had been before this moment and everything they would become beyond it.

My heart was pounding and my head started to bang, as if I could actually feel and hear the blood rushing around it. This was all just too much. I'd known it was possible that this was what he was going to say, but as long as there was one fraction of hope that he might be able to tell us it was something else entirely, I was going to cling to it. Now this doctor, with all his years of training and experience, was saying this really was Alzheimer's.

This was it. No doubt. It was happening all over again – but this time it was happening to me.

I think the doctor must have left the room for a bit then. When he came back, he carried on talking, saying he understood what a shock this would be, that we could meet again when we were ready to discuss the next steps, reassuring us it was very early-onset dementia and lots and lots and lots more words that I didn't really hear amid the deafening roar in my head: *I have Alzheimer's and it's never going away.*

Martin spoke first. 'OK, right . . . Well, we will need a bit of time to digest this.'

'Of course, of course,' replied the doctor.

I didn't say anything. There was nothing to say. I looked from Martin to the doctor and back again as I felt my entire life seep away in this little office with the traffic roaring outside and people bustling up and down corridors, without their lives having just been shredded.

I'm told the doctor said we should go home and try to live 'as normally as possible', but that they would continue to monitor my progress. I think I must have missed that, though, or maybe I completely forgot about it.

Martin and I must have got up and left the office, trooped down the stairs and out onto the street below although I don't really remember any of that. It was all just a blur.

I'd only turned sixty-one at the start of that year. And, while I suppose I had always thought I might get the disease one day, I'd hoped it might be when I was in my eighties or even nineties. I didn't think that 'one day' would be 'today' – but I guess no one ever does.

We stood on the pavement outside the hospital in complete and utter shock. Then Martin said: 'Right, well, shall we go and have a drink?'

'Yes, let's,' I replied. 'I think I need a drink.'

We walked across the road to a little pub called the Queen's Larder on the opposite side of the square from the hospital, both too shell-shocked to speak much. Martin went to the bar for two large glasses of wine while I sat at a table, fiddling with a bar mat and listening to two old blokes discussing football while my life continued to shatter into a million shards of pain.

In those first few minutes after the devastating diagnosis, I was angry too. Really fucking angry. So, after everything I had been through, after all the worry of looking after Mum as she became lost in her confusion and terror and then the heartache of seeing my independent dad have his personality stripped away from him, now it was coming for me. I know you're not supposed to ask 'Why me?' – and I've never been a moaner – but seriously, this time, 'Why me?' What had I done so wrong to deserve this? It's not like I needed any more lessons in quite how awful this illness can be, I could write a whole book. In fact, I *had* written the book ten years earlier. If it wasn't so bloody awful, it would be funny.

Martin brought the drinks over and we sat there trying to make sense of what the doctor had just told us. He was so pale, so utterly shocked.

'What do we do now?' I asked.

He probably hadn't any more idea than me but, despite years and years of independence and not feeling I needed anyone to cope, I really needed to cling to him at that moment.

'Well, the consultant told us to go home and live as "normally" as we can,' Martin said flatly.

'How on earth do we live "normally"?' I asked.

'I'm not sure,' he replied. 'We'll just have to give it a go and see what treatments we can find. There must be something we can do. I'll talk to some experts and see what they say. There's so much work going on in this field nowadays, it really has progressed enormously since your mum was ill.'

I knew Martin had flipped into journalist mode – as if he was editing a news show and a bomb had just gone off or a major celebrity had died: 'OK, right, this has happened. What do we need to do next? Who do we need to speak to? Where do we need to send reporters?' It was like that – this wasn't the time to flap or fuss, we just had to get the job done. And I liked that. Because if anyone knew what to do in a crisis it was Martin.

I just felt floored. Like I'd taken one enormous great sucker punch to my gut and I was never getting up. And as for going home to live as 'normally as possible', how was that possible? Nothing would ever be normal again. And yet as we sat there in that pub, it was entirely normal. The lovely landlady collected glasses and wiped tables, some office workers came in and had two pints of Guinness, the television in the corner was showing the news. It felt like everything for everyone was just carrying on the same.

Everyone except me.

Martin and I made a pact that day that we wouldn't tell anyone what the consultant had said.

'I don't want anyone finding out, Martin,' I said. 'And I mean anyone. I don't want the boys knowing yet as it will only worry them and I don't want them going through the worry I went through with my mum. And I don't want them pussyfooting around me or feeling embarrassed to bring their friends home because their mum's going mad. And I don't want people peering at me in the streets every time I go to the shop.'

I was having none of that.

So we did as the consultant had suggested, but which had seemed utterly impossible: we went home and lived 'as normally as possible'. I think we both realized that in reality, it's difficult to do anything other than 'normal' – you are hard-wired to it.

The next morning Martin got up to go to work, just as he always did. I got up and made a coffee then went for a walk, just as I always did. What else could we do? Lie on the floor, weeping and wailing? That certainly wasn't going to change anything. We both had sleepless nights in the weeks that followed, but each morning we would get up and try to make the best of things. And over the next few days and weeks, I could sometimes go for long periods not thinking about my diagnosis at all, but then the realization of what it meant would sweep over me like a tsunami. And the anger came in waves too – the rage that I'd been chosen for this disease.

We stuck to our vow of not telling the boys and I think I was able to hide it from them quite well. Martin says I would forget things and they must have noticed there were changes in my behaviour, but it wasn't like I was doing anything really strange. Or not that I was aware of.

I was determined to keep the diagnosis a very tight secret. That for me was very important. When you have been forced to live a lot of your life in public by being on television, you become very conscious about which parts you want to keep for yourself. And I couldn't bear to be judged by people for having Alzheimer's. Oh, I know no one would ever admit to judging someone like me, but I saw it for myself when I was caring for Mum and Dad. People do judge, they whisper behind their hands or try to avoid someone who is struggling. I hated the thought of becoming an object of gossip or even pity.

I could imagine in the world of TV some of those people I used to work with saying, 'Oh, have you heard about poor Fiona? What a tragedy!' I'd worked so hard to be independent and judged on my own merits, so the thought now of people patronizing me like that was too awful. I just had to keep plodding along in the way we always had for as long as we could.

That afternoon in the pub it had seemed extraordinary that we could continue to live life 'as normally as possible', but that's exactly what we did from that moment on. We drove down the road we had driven down a million times before, opened the door to the home where we had brought up our boys, then sat in the front room and watched TV. Nat was away in the army, Mackenzie was out with his mates. Everything was normal. But then what was our alternative?

There was no Plan B.

This was my life now.

25

Martin

In the final few weeks before Fiona's diagnosis, I had feared this was what the doctor was going to say. And, like Fiona, I was delighted when the consultant said her spinal fluid was 'good' and 'clear'. It was only later we found out that what he had actually meant was that a clear sample was easier to test; the clearness didn't have any impact on what the results might be. But, in those weeks while we waited, we clung to that one sentence and the possibility that this wasn't Alzheimer's after all and that Fiona could have something else entirely, something treatable.

Fiona's mood was suddenly so much lighter. She was like a teenager again, utterly transformed by relief. I tried to be the voice of caution and said: 'Well, let's just wait until the results come back,' but she was convinced she hadn't got it and everything was going to be OK.

We had a whole month before the test results were due back. In many ways it was a wonderful time. We spent two weeks in Italy and it was like all this had never happened. Even the symptoms went away. Fiona wasn't depressed, she was happy to go out for dinner in the evenings. She remembered everything. She was carefree, laughing, joking, chatting to me about things we could do when we got home. It was amazing! She was like the old Fiona again. No, what I mean is she was like the *young* Fiona again. For the first time in ages, everything seemed good. I still thought there was a strong chance that it was Alzheimer's because there would still be moments of memory lapse. That's why I didn't want Fiona getting too hopeful, but her behaviour had changed so much that even I was holding out hope that maybe it was just the menopause or something else and she was coming through it.

She really believed she was getting better because she felt better. I guess that shows how much the depression she had been suffering had been caused, quite naturally, by the fear of what was awaiting her.

We'd only been back from holiday for a couple of days when it was time to get the test results. On the way to the hospital that morning, the nerves were back in full force.

We went up to the consultant's room and sat down in front of him at his desk. He had a pile of documents in front of him with graphs and charts and all the results from Fiona's tests. And then there was that moment that Fiona has described when he looked up at us and said: 'I'm afraid to tell you that you do have early-onset Alzheimer's disease.'

The silence was total. It was an absence of noise, but also an absence of everything. There was nothing to say. Nothing that could comfort Fiona, because she knew exactly what this meant.

There was no funny line to make this go away, nothing smart to say.

Nothing.

And then the doctor said he'd leave us in the room alone for a bit to digest it all.

'I'll get you both a cup of tea and here's some things to look at while I'm doing that.'

And then, God bless him, he pushed some leaflets across the desk. On the cover of one of them was a picture of a couple of eighty-somethings with walking sticks and grey hair and glasses, holding onto each other outside a care home. That wasn't us. Fiona had just turned sixty-one. She was wearing skinny jeans and high-heeled boots. This was a degenerative disease for old people like the ones on the leaflet – it shouldn't be happening to someone as young as Fiona.

It was utterly gut-wrenching. Sickening. We just looked at each other.

Shit! What are we going to do now?

I'd sort of known this was coming, but to actually hear those words from the mouth of an expert was a totally different thing. There was no room for even a sliver of doubt now. This was it, our fate had been decided and it was real. But the worst thing was seeing how utterly shocked Fiona was; she was completely floored. On one level, Fiona knew that she'd been given a death sentence, on another level I don't think she was able to fully understand the ramifications. It was all too much for her to absorb in the moment.

I didn't say anything to Fiona that day, but there was another fear lurking in the back of my mind: if she had inherited the disease from her parents and grandmother, did that mean our boys might have inherited this family curse too? The thought that these strong young men with their entire lives in front of them might also be facing this death sentence was horrendous – and another reason we couldn't tell them what was happening.

Not yet.

26

Fiona

———

In the months that followed, there were frequent trips back and forth to the hospital. After each trip Martin and I got into the habit of popping into the Queen's Larder pub near the hospital, where we had gone for a drink the day of my diagnosis. It's a beautiful old-fashioned wood-panelled place and must be the last pub in London still serving Spam fritters! Some of the locals recognized me — they must have been *GMTV* fans back in the day. They were always so lovely and we'd have great chats. After another morning of gloomy news at the hospital it would lift my spirits so much to have a laugh with them — it became a refuge.

Martin and I were determined to find any possible treatment for my illness. He spent hours googling new research and then, during one of our meetings with the consultant at UCLH at the start of 2023, it was suggested that I might be eligible to take part in trials they were doing on a new drug to slow the advancement of Alzheimer's and maybe even reverse it altogether.

The trial was about to start and they had almost filled all the slots, but they still needed one or two more people to make up the quota of volunteers. There was no guarantee that I would be eligible, though, as for the trials to work you have to be at a particular stage of the disease – not too early but not too late either.

To check whether I was suitable and that my condition was still just mild Alzheimer's and not too advanced, I had to go through a whole series of tests. It was like the questions they had asked when I first went for tests, but this time it was even more terrifying as I so wanted to be selected to try the new drug. They'd ask me questions like 'Which month is it?', 'What season is it?' and then a whole load more of those subtraction questions. It felt like being back in school – and not in a good way when we were laughing and messing around at the back of the class at Millbrook School. This was stressful and I knew it was so important to get the questions right, but beforehand I'd be thinking, *Oh God, what if I don't know the answers or I do know the answers but I get too nervous?* I was absolutely desperate to be chosen to trial this new drug.

After completing the tests there were then another couple of weeks of waiting and doing that 'living as normally as possible' thing we'd been told to do. I invested all my hope in being accepted onto the trials; I talked to Martin about them all the time, desperate to be chosen. It felt like my only escape route from this terrible situation.

When they called us back to the hospital to say I'd passed the tests, I was beyond delighted. It was just in the nick of time too – I was the last person accepted for it. Now there was something to hope for again. Maybe this drug could be the miracle that for hundreds of years people had been waiting for.

After more tests to show I was physically fit and healthy, the doctors sent us home with an enormous bag of paraphernalia for administering the drug. There were tiny syringes and phials of drugs that had to be administered three times a day.

Martin would do the first injection before he went to work in the morning then do another as soon as he got in the door from work in the late afternoon and then a final one before bed. They all went into my stomach and my poor tummy soon looked like a pin cushion – he was literally stabbing me morning, noon and night.

For the trial to work, half of us guinea pigs were on the actual new drug they hoped would slow Alzheimer's while the other half were on a placebo – basically just water or something that would make no difference at all to the condition. The idea was that by having half the triallists on a fake drug – or control – they would be able to see the differences in how a patient's condition develops.

I spent a lot of time wondering if I was on the real drug or the fake one, but there was no way of finding out. The packaging for all the triallists was exactly the same. And even the doctors themselves who handed the drugs out at UCLH didn't know – only the scientists in the lab would know when they got the results in.

I certainly felt OK during those first few months, although I got pretty sick of the injections – I just hoped against hope that the reason I felt OK was down to the miracle drug. I don't think I believed I would be cured, but perhaps the illness could be slowed in its tracks. Otherwise I was quite healthy and living a good life, so if the choice was that the illness would just hang around at the back of my head without getting any worse, I'd have taken that option all day long.

That's what I had to hope for.

The doctors had also prescribed me donepezil, which is sold under the name Aricept and has been used for years to treat Alzheimer's. It can't stop the disease, but it can slow it down in some people. I wasn't massively convinced it would make much difference, though – as I've said, Mum had been on exactly the same medication twenty years earlier and it hadn't done much for her. I took it nevertheless, but all my real hope was focused on my three-times-a-day injections.

I was also prescribed an antidepressant – sertraline – to help with the anxiety and weepiness I'd been feeling. I still don't know if the depression was a side effect of my Alzheimer's or if it came with the dawning realization of what was happening to me. Either way, I took the tablets as instructed.

The three-times-a-day injections continued for a year. And apart from the endless stabbings to the stomach, we just got on with normal life. Or as normal as it could be.

Sometimes I would meet my friend Amanda for coffee. There's a lovely coffee shop at the end of my road, which was my regular haunt. They knew my favourite drink – an oat-milk latte – and if I did forget things or became confused about the menu, which I don't think happened very often, they were understanding. Amanda and I would chat about how our children were getting on and the daily events of life, but I didn't tell her about my diagnosis – I just couldn't face it. When we were together I preferred being able to avoid thinking about it, chatting the way we always had done.

That summer of 2023, Martin and I were invited to watch the Grand Prix and we had a wonderful day out. I've always loved cars and the thrill of racing. That and the free champagne in the sunshine make for a great day out! Out and about, I could chat to anyone without them thinking anything was happening to me.

We also went to the Pride of Britain Awards, which is always such a lovely evening with so many celebrities I'd known for years, as well as inspirational winners who just kept going in their lives, no matter what was thrown at them – I hoped I could be like that.

We even managed to get in a couple of short breaks to Italy, which I loved. It was so quiet and peaceful and I could sit in the shade and watch the world go by.

Perfect.

In comparison, London felt very busy and noisy.

But despite me trying to tell you about the positive moments during that time, there were some dark days too. Around then the doctors also advised that I should stop driving, just in case I hurt myself or someone else, though it barely registered with me. I'd not been behind the wheel for months as I found the speed and stress of the roads too overwhelming. It was quite strange that after all those years of feeling so independent in my car – even bombing along the freeways in LA – I had barely noticed my little Mini for a while, as it sat untouched outside the front of our house, looking a bit dusty and sad. Neither Martin nor I could face selling it, though – that felt a bit final. After a while, as with so many other things, I just forgot that I didn't drive any more – it became another part of my new normal.

But I also couldn't face the thought of being all squashed up with thousands of other people on the tube. Crowds terrified me. And it wasn't like I was desperate to get anywhere. If I wanted to go further afield – to get my hair cut or wander around the shops – I would take the bus as I knew where to get on and off and it wasn't too busy. But most of all I preferred staying closer to home and was happy to walk wherever I needed to get to.

My lack of interest in food continued too. I couldn't face cooking any more, so Martin would make something when he got in from work that I might pick at. I'd never had an enormous appetite, but now it was less than ever. There were times around then when I would get very low if I thought too much about what was happening and the thing that was most upsetting – and still is – was that I couldn't get out to work. I didn't feel confident enough to take on any more TV work and whenever I tried to sit down and write my *Mirror* column, I just couldn't find the right idea or the right words. My contract was allowed to lapse on the promise that I would return when I felt up to it. I couldn't bring myself to tell them that might never happen.

I've tried to explain in this book over and over again how important work was to me, how much it was part of my identity. And it wasn't to do with the money or the status or any of that – I just felt by working I was being me. Without work, I didn't feel like me.

Some days I'd wake up and think, *Maybe I'll try this today or maybe I'll do that*, but then the day went on and I never quite got it together. Other times I would wake and not be able to face walking round the same streets or going to the same old places for a cup of coffee – it all felt pointless. The doctors said feeling depressed was a very common side effect of Alzheimer's and let's face it, there's plenty to be depressed about. The anti-depressants probably stabilized me a bit – it felt like they enabled me to sometimes forget what was going on. And I really did try not to moan on all the time, not that Martin would have noticed!

I put on a brave face if I met a friend for coffee or when the boys came in from work – I didn't want to drag everyone else down with me. But I was different with Martin, I guess. He more than anyone saw the real me and would get the full download each evening of how I was feeling.

Martin got me at my lowest and moaniest and for that – and everything else – I appreciated him in a way I don't think I had ever done before. He was absolutely dedicated to giving me the injections and making sure he was with me at every single hospital appointment. He'd always been incredibly patient with me throughout our marriage – when I was rushing out in the morning to go to work, leaving him with the kids, when I was very low during those final days at *GMTV* and keeping everything going at home when I was caring for my parents. He'd always been a good husband, but this was something else. He was still working – he had to work to pay the bills, and he loved work. But he still managed to make me feel entirely supported too.

27

Martin

———————

From the moment Fiona was given her diagnosis, she handed over total responsibility for her treatment to me. She didn't want to talk about it; she didn't want to engage with it at all. She was – and sometimes still is – in a state of denial about what was happening to her. That's why she found this part of the book so difficult to write and entrusted more of it to me and Alison Phillips. Maybe a symptom of the illness is that she isn't able to think about what is happening to her. But not once post-diagnosis did she say, 'I've been looking things up and I think I should try this' or 'What about if I tried that treatment or drug?' Even though, at that time, she still had the cognitive ability to do that kind of research and was capable of that kind of thinking, she just didn't want to go there.

A couple of weeks before the diagnosis, we had been in Italy talking about politics and the news and whatever else couples chat about, so she was mentally alert in many ways, but when it came to researching or thinking about her own condition there was a total block. As I've said, she was totally in denial.

This might sound very strange, or maybe not to other couples going through this, but we have not once discussed her illness since her diagnosis. Never. Obviously, we have both been in the room when the doctors are talking to us both about how she's getting on and we have discussed the logistics of administering her injections and tablets; we have also worked together shaping this book – but writing it down is easier than talking it through step by step. The big issues around what is happening to her – and what will happen next – we have left untouched.

Fiona doesn't want to talk about it, she doesn't really want to accept it exists. Even in creating this book she finds it easier to talk about her day-to-day experiences than the bigger picture. And, really, where's the benefit in us talking about it? I mean we have planned together around the practical things such as getting our finances in order and family paperwork so everything is sorted for the future, but then it's really a case of 'let's just wait for it to come'. Talking about what is happening to her isn't going to make Fiona feel better. This isn't someone who has an illness where talking therapy might help, because she would only forget the conversation anyway. Besides, she finds any mention of it upsetting and so we get on with life around the edges of what is happening.

We did tackle one fear and talked to Fiona's consultant about whether she had inherited the illness from her parents.

He said: 'We suggest Fiona has a genetic test, because if this has come down through your family there is a danger that your children may have it too, in which case they might have to think about IVF if they want to have children. That would be a big decision for them, but screening embryos for the gene would break the lineage. And, of course, they will have to be told.'

That was an awful thought. The boys were still only in their early twenties, they were just starting out in life and it would be horrendous to have this hanging over them from then on. And they weren't even approaching the point in their lives when they were thinking about children. It was a lot to deal with, but we knew we had to find out.

Two weeks after Fiona's diagnosis, she returned for the genetic blood testing and, once again, we were left waiting to learn our family's fate. Thankfully, when we were called back in for the results, the doctor said the test had come back negative.

'Fiona is clearly predisposed to the illness,' the consultant said. 'But it is not genetic – she doesn't carry a particular gene that meant she would inevitably get it. And so that means the boys won't carry that gene either.'

'Oh, right,' I said.

I didn't entirely understand what he meant. How could someone be 'predisposed' to a particular disease if there wasn't something in their genetic make-up that determined it? But he assured me this was the case. While Fiona's chances of getting the disease had always been a lot higher, that didn't mean she would pass it on to her children. And, when I researched it, it appeared that this is the case in other families too. The most famous case is actor Chris Hemsworth, who played Thor in the

Marvel movies. He doesn't have Alzheimer's, but he has been found to be predisposed to it, so there's a greater chance he might get it at some point compared with other people. As a result, he has been cutting back on his film work so he can enjoy what time he does have, in case he does start to lose his memory in the years to come.

At a time when there really wasn't much good news in our lives, the thought that our boys might dodge the illness because they didn't carry a particular gene came as an enormous relief. Also, there was no history of the disease on my side of the family.

A few months later we told the boys what was happening. By then, they were aware on some level that something was not right with their mum. She was even more withdrawn and forgetful and they knew she'd had a series of hospital appointments. Rather than it being one big moment with us all sat around the table and the terrible news landing on them like a bomb, I'd gradually shared with them the sense that something was very wrong. When the moment came and I used the dreaded 'Alzheimer's' word, I think they were prepared for it – however awful that news was. At least we could tell them that there was no genetic link, which was a small relief. But mostly they were just heartbroken for their mum, though she didn't want to make a big fuss about it all. She was able to dismiss it from her mind and so the conversation quickly moved on. It may sound strange, but that is how it was. Even though she was suffering herself, I think she was determined to protect the boys from worrying about her. They'd been very little when their grandparents were ill with the disease, but they could still remember how awful it was.

There wasn't one moment when everything changed at home. Fiona was still able to potter round, tidy up and sometimes prepare food. She didn't need to be cared for and still protected her independence, going out for walks, meeting friends and popping out to the shops. The anxiety was still there, but she coped; we coped. For a fair while, things just rolled on pretty much the way they had over the previous few years.

And to people who met Fiona in the street, she probably seemed pretty much the same. We would often go for breakfast on a Saturday morning and she would chat to the waiters or anyone in the cafe and no one would have thought she had a care in the world.

Sometimes I wonder if she was well-practised at putting on that cheerful mask after years of working in television, where she had to keep on smiling even when someone (often me!) was yelling in her earpiece that the next segment was being pulled and everything was going to hell. I don't know whether it was a conscious or subconscious thing but Fiona was still able to put on a great show in public. At home, though, the periods of forgetfulness continued and she found that distressing.

The one hope was that we might be able to enrol Fiona on an Alzheimer's drugs trial taking place at the tiny, charity-funded Leonard Wolfson unit at the Royal Neurological Hospital, part of UCLH.

Fiona is right to say that when she was initially diagnosed,

I probably took a very journalistic approach to dealing with a crisis – 'OK, this is the problem. Now, how are we going to fix it?' I did hours and hours of research online and quickly discovered that in the hundred years or so since Alzheimer's was first diagnosed, nothing much had moved on.

I'd been aware of Alzheimer's obviously because of what it did to Fiona's parents, but like many people I was guilty of thinking of it only as an old person's disease. Amy, Fiona's mum, had actually been quite young when she got it, but by the time I met her, she seemed old. I just thought maybe she was incredibly unlucky and she lived in far west Wales where perhaps they didn't have the best medical resources or awareness of the disease – I never once thought that little would have changed in terms of treatment when Fiona was diagnosed.

Even those cognitive tests sufferers have to do, which give them a score determining if they have totally lost it or are actually completely compos mentis, are the same tests that were developed fifty years ago. It seemed very little had moved on in this field for years, but now we were on the cusp of lots of research coming through. The worry was whether that research would translate into publicly available drugs in time to help Fiona.

Spending so much time on Google also confirmed what I had already known – that for someone like Fiona, diagnosed with Alzheimer's at an early age, life expectancy would be a lot shorter than for someone who contracted it later in life. That was horrible, and made me not want to think about how long she might have had it, because that would reduce the time we might have left.

Fiona is an extremely smart woman who has been an ambassador for the Alzheimer's Society so she would have known what the prognosis would be for people with early onset of the disease. At that point she still had the capability to consider that sort of thing – I just think she couldn't face it.

And I was the same in many ways.

Rather than consider the future, I just wanted to do everything I could to try to fix the issue. Not that there was a fix, but doing something was better than feeling helpless.

So I talked to the doctors and it was then that they said they were still looking for participants for the drugs trial. I was determined Fiona should get on it – it felt like our only hope.

What was particularly exciting about the research on this drug was that this was the third year of the trial. Previous years had already convinced the scientists that the drugs could deliver results for people with Alzheimer's. This third year of testing mainly focused on if there were any side effects or safety issues. It seemed like an amazing opportunity to get treated with this groundbreaking drug that might not be available more widely for at least a couple of years – and then only if it received the funding to be administered. Quite often drugs are available that could help people, but they are deemed too expensive by NICE (the National Institute for Health and Care Excellence, the body that regulates which drugs are available in the UK).

But, before we could get anywhere near the hoped-for new drug, Fiona had to pass all the tests she has talked about. That meant more trips back and forward to the hospital while they assessed her suitability. What was crucial, I felt, was for us to show that her condition wasn't too far advanced. Even though I knew she was frequently forgetting things and repeating herself, there were other times when she was still very sparky with an extensive vocabulary and able to remember specific incidents from years before. I was determined she gave a good show of herself in the tests.

In a taxi on the way to one of the tests, I found myself drumming the answers into her, as if I was helping a kid cram up before a GCSE in ten minutes' time. 'OK, Fiona,' I said. 'If they ask the month, remember it's March. If they ask the date, it's the 22nd. The season is spring and if they ask how old you are, you're sixty-two.'

Looking back, my coaching was probably utterly pointless because she was either able to remember what month it was or she wasn't – revising really wasn't going to make any difference.

A couple of weeks after that, we were told Fiona had been accepted – she was on the drugs trial. But there were still weeks and weeks of waiting and further tests before things properly got underway.

Every time we went to the hospital, I'd thank the doctors for accepting Fiona onto the trials – it felt like they had thrown us a lifeline. But they were just as grateful to us, which seemed strange. They explained that lots of people are so traumatized once they receive an Alzheimer's diagnosis that they can't face being part of a drugs trial programme – they just think any treatment is pointless and want to turn away from the world.

To be accepted onto the trial the sufferer also had to have a partner or buddy who agreed to attend every hospital appointment with them – of which there were loads. That person also had to be there to administer the drug three times a day, which is done with a tiny syringe. It couldn't be left to the sufferer themselves in case they got confused about doses. For the scientific research to be robust, the rules of taking the drugs had to be followed to the letter, but that is a big time commitment, so I guess many people, particularly if they were older or living alone, weren't able to volunteer for the trials.

As Fiona has explained, I had to administer the drug through a syringe into her belly three times a day – for a year. I'm genuinely astonished I was able to do it, being most definitely a sufferer of 'white coat syndrome'. Not only do I have a loathing of visiting a hospital or anywhere that mortality might be played out, the sight of blood, needles, monitors and even trolleys can all make me lightheaded. Taking my blood pressure is an almost impossible task for a nurse as my readings go shooting through the roof! However, who was I to be squeamish when Fiona had no future to look forward to? I got on and did the jabs. The trial drug, devised by a British scientist, was aimed at preventing the growth of platelets that originate in the liver long before they get the chance to smother the brain – at least that's the layman's version of it – and this explained why the injections were centred on Fiona's midriff.

It was only a very tiny needle so I don't think it particularly hurt her, but it was still a gruelling regime that we had to stick to, come hell or high water. Over the weeks that passed, I watched Fiona like a hawk to see if there was any change in her behaviour. Not knowing if she was on the actual drug or a placebo became like a game of spot the difference to see if she appeared to be stabilizing – or even getting better.

At first it was hard to tell. She was still having moments of forgetfulness and memory lapse. She would forget her mobile phone if she went out or if I asked her if she'd eaten any lunch that day then she wouldn't remember. If a friend came round and asked out of politeness what we had done at the weekend, she wouldn't be able to tell them, but then in the next breath she might be talking about Boris Johnson or whatever the latest TV scandal was – so she did do an amazing job at hiding what was going on.

We went to Italy again and she seemed great when we were there. It was a very familiar environment for her because we had been going there for years and she seemed calm, which made her memory better. I guess during that period we were both coming to terms with our new reality. Fiona was incredibly accepting of what was happening and quite quickly I realized that I had to be the same. Neither of us was going to be able to stop what was happening, but at least we could try to do everything in our power to slow it.

After her initial rage, Fiona never said: 'Why me?' And I didn't either. In fact, every time we went for more tests or results at UCLH, I simply felt enormously grateful that we had been given a strand of hope to cling to at a place that is right at the cutting edge of research into this illness. There are so many different projects going on there that will make a huge difference to lives in the future. It definitely helped both of us to be close to that environment in those months following Fiona's diagnosis.

Even if Fiona was only on a placebo rather than the trial drug, it did help her. And even if she was on the real thing and there was some terrible side effect we didn't yet know about, we didn't mind. Because just being on that drug trial and feeling we were part of something that might help slow the disease was incredibly helpful. A doctor told me that one of the most effective treatments they'd ever trialled at the hospital was the placebo – the injection that actually contained no drug. That was because the effect of thinking they might be on the treatment had given sufferers a sense of hope. That lifted their natural 'happy hormone' serotonin levels, which in turn helped fight the disease. So, either way, if Fiona was on the real drug or the placebo, there was a benefit.

After about four months I thought I could see a change in Fiona. I wasn't sure if this was just wishful thinking on my part and maybe I was too close to know for certain, but she seemed less anxious. And while there were still episodes of forgetfulness, she generally had a clearer mind and could be engaged in conversations going on around her. Her condition seemed to have plateaued and definitely wasn't getting worse, as had been happening before the trials. She was less depressed, more with it. And crucially, more wanting to be with it – the hopelessness that had plagued her for years seemed to be waning.

We knew the trial would only last a year and time was racing by. All we could do was take the benefits that it seemed to be offering while they lasted.

28

Fiona

———

My favourite place to go at the time was the little cafe at the end of our road for a slice of their amazing toasted banana bread and an oat milk latte. I would sometimes meet up there with a friend from the *Mirror*. I was so determined to keep what was happening to me secret that I didn't even tell my best friend, Amanda, who I would still meet most weeks too. I became paranoid that if I told even one person, they might tell someone else who might tell someone else and, before I knew it, I'd be on the cover of a women's magazine again.

Martin once said to me: 'I think Amanda will already know.'

'How?' I said. 'I haven't said anything about it and she hasn't mentioned anything either.'

'But she will know,' he insisted. 'Because your behaviour has changed – sometimes you repeat yourself or you forget things when you go out for a coffee.'

We had that conversation several times, but I wasn't convinced.

'Just because your friend might be a bit confused one day I don't think you'd automatically assume she has Alzheimer's,' I snapped.

'But she knows you well enough and meets you often enough,' Martin told me.

Sometimes he really can't let something go. But then neither can I. Anyway, even if Amanda did know something, she hadn't said anything to me and I still didn't want our nice chats over coffee to be destroyed by me having to drone on about my illness every time we met.

Apart from family and my close friends, I guess the staff in that cafe saw me more frequently than anyone. Did they think sometimes my behaviour was a little odd? If I'd gone out without my purse or put my mobile phone down and couldn't find it? Or couldn't read the menu because I didn't have my glasses? Or sometimes just got a little lost with the menu and found it slightly overwhelming? I don't know. But the waitresses were very patient with me and would point me in the right direction if occasionally I couldn't remember the way to the toilet, even though I'd been there many times before. But I don't think they would have thought there was anything clinically wrong with me. It wasn't as if I was going round with a big sign over my head saying: 'I've got Alzheimer's' and for a long while that's exactly how I wanted it to stay.

But gradually Martin and I thought maybe I should start telling more people. Martin felt that if more people knew what was happening to me then they wouldn't judge me if I did ever start behaving unusually – not that I thought I did. It was hardly like I was going down the street half-clothed, yelling at people. But he and the doctors, who I was constantly backwards and forwards to see, would say that I kept repeating myself and that sometimes I forgot what I was doing or where I was going.

The strange thing was I had no awareness of that.

Martin kept reassuring me that there was nothing to be embarrassed about when it came to making my diagnosis public. He'd say, 'It's not like you've done anything wrong or you have anything to be ashamed about. You've been diagnosed with an illness that impacts millions of people across the country and people will be inspired by your honesty; they're not going to pity you.'

That was my major concern. I'd probably inherited it from Dad, but I hated the idea of being pitied: 'Oh, look at poor old Fiona in the corner,' I could imagine people saying. It made me feel sick.

I guess after all the work I had done when Mum and Dad were ill to raise awareness about Alzheimer's and the need for research into a cure, it made perfect sense that I should be open about what was happening to me now. But I was still wary of what people would say and whether they would judge me, particularly if it meant I never got offered work again. I was still desperate to get back to work, I just needed to feel a bit more myself first.

In the end, I agreed to do it: I would tell people I had this illness. As I'd worked for the *Mirror* writing my column for more than twenty years, it made perfect sense that I should tell my story to them. Martin and I discussed it over and over and he suggested I should call Alison Phillips, who was then-editor of the *Mirror*, to explain why I had been unable to write my column for so long – and to tell my readers what had happened too.

Alison agreed to meet Martin and me for lunch and we told her how my fears about the menopause had worsened and now I'd had this awful diagnosis. She had interviewed me many times in the past and it almost seemed like I was telling the next instalment in my family's story.

When you are a journalist yourself it is strange being interviewed. You are so used to being the one asking the questions that it feels a bit unnerving being on the other end of things. But when I was working on *GMTV* there was nothing I hated more than people who came on the show and agreed to be interviewed, then dodged questions or were clearly giving an overly rehearsed anodyne answer rather than actually saying what they really felt. I would never be that person so whatever the questions were, I did try my hardest to answer them honestly.

Maybe the toughest one was when Alison asked: 'Do you ever find, Fiona, there are times when, because of the illness, you forget that you have it?'

That was hard to answer because, in truth, I wasn't entirely sure. How can you remember whether you have forgotten something? Although I guess we all do at times, don't we?

'Mmm, yes, I think so,' I replied.

'And so does that bring you moments of peace, where you're not having to worry about the illness if you forget about having it?' she asked.

'I don't really like having too much time to myself,' I replied. 'I never have done – I love working so not working has left a big hole in my life. But there are times when I'm at home and I don't feel anxious or anything. I'm just quite content sitting there.'

As the interview went on, Alison asked if I felt I'd been carrying around a huge burden by keeping my illness secret. I'd not really thought of it like that before.

'It's a horrible bloody secret to divulge to anyone,' I said. 'I don't want to make a big thing of it because I do still think people put labels on people with this illness. And the reality is no one has ever been cured of Alzheimer's. There is no cure and that's the awful thing.'

I wasn't going to hide from the awfulness of what was happening to me, but I didn't want to wallow in self-pity either. And I was very keen to make the point that this whole interview wasn't about me wanting to talk about myself – I only wanted to use my experience in some way to help others who were suffering as a result of Alzheimer's.

I hoped that because I was still relatively young and physically fit and healthy myself then it might change some of those perceptions that exist about Alzheimer's being an old person's disease. I was the living proof, if anyone wanted it (which they don't!), that this disease can strike anyone at any time and crucially we need the research and drugs to fight it.

For years, if Martin and I were out, people would frequently come up to me in the street and thank me for everything I had done to raise awareness of Alzheimer's after my parents died. Often they were very emotional and I could tell many of them were desperately upset by the effect the disease had had on their family. I was conscious that I needed to try to help those people in some way – and the millions more who will still be impacted by the illness in years to come. Now I felt I had the chance to amplify all those people's experiences and to finally ensure Alzheimer's disease got the attention it deserved.

Around about then there had also been a lot of publicity about the *Die Hard* actor Bruce Willis, who had been diagnosed at the age of sixty-seven with frontotemporal dementia (FTD), a rare form of dementia that affects a different part of the brain to Alzheimer's, causing emotional problems, difficulty finding the right words to communicate and struggles with walking and movement. And there had been publicity too, as we've mentioned earlier, about Chris Hemsworth's decision to take time out from acting because of his warning that he had a higher chance of developing dementia.

I was hoping that maybe I could make a TV project interviewing people like Bruce Willis and Chris Hemsworth about their experiences once I'd explained to the public what was happening to me. And I wanted to talk to people with Alzheimer's from across the UK – and their families – about what support they needed. The difficult thing with this illness is by the time it becomes so noticeable that people want to share their experiences, they have often reached a point where it is too difficult for them to do so.

As I said in the *Mirror* interview: 'There are so many people suffering around the world – and so many others who may not even know they are in the early stages of Alzheimer's. I just want to do everything I can to make it something that people are more prepared to talk about and, crucially, something people seek help for as early as possible.'

Martin helped me during the interview as there were parts of my story around how I had increasingly become confused in certain situations that I didn't know about myself. Sometimes I needed him to be there to give his perspective on what I had been saying and doing. Not that I always agreed with him – no chance!

Martin told Alison that what had begun as a struggle coping with the enormity of the diagnosis had slipped into clinical depression. I was quite surprised.

'Do you think so?' I asked. 'I don't really think I have been very depressed.'

'Oh, Fiona, you have,' he replied, smiling at me.

And once again I did feel genuinely confused.

'Well, I'm trying not to be depressed,' I snapped.

We talked too about how there were gaps in my recollections. I knew from all the previous research I'd done into Alzheimer's that someone suffering from it was more able to remember events from the past than they were things that had happened recently – I just wasn't sure that applied to me yet.

'But you do struggle with remembering details about how you were diagnosed and how we have got to this point after the past few years,' Martin insisted.

'How does that make you feel?' Alison said. 'How does it make you feel when Martin says he thinks there are gaps in your recollections?'

'It's really weird because I didn't think there was anything wrong with me,' I said. 'And I don't want to make this a big thing and make this "Me".'

'But you're not surprised by my saying there are clear gaps, are you, Fiona?' said Martin gently, 'Because this is what the symptoms are.'

'I know,' I replied. 'I know.'

And I did know. I *do* know. I know exactly what the symptoms are and what the prognosis is, but at the same time I could not know it was happening to me. 'I just can't believe it is here,' I said.

It's so hard to explain.

As we chatted that long afternoon over lunch and then endless cups of tea, I found myself more able to express how I'd really been feeling. At that point I was more able to articulate how I felt at times and where my real anxieties lay. I recalled how Alzheimer's had impacted Mum's life. But maybe I wasn't really just talking about Mum – maybe I was talking about my own fears for my future too.

Martin had asked me as we chatted: 'When did you notice your mum was unwell?'

'She was crying all the time and she got lost,' I said. 'That's so awful – if you get lost and you can't make yourself known, and you are frightened and you are crying and you are all alone. That happens a lot to people with this illness. So . . .'

Alison was clearly trying to reassure me when she said: 'Well, that may happen to some people with the illness, but it won't necessarily happen to you.'

'Yeah,' I replied, not entirely convinced. 'I just can't believe any of this is happening to me and that we are sitting here talking about this, although it was clearly there lying in wait for me all the time. All those graves of my family with "Alzheimer's" on the headstone.'

As the interview went on, I was finally able to talk about how depressed the diagnosis had made me feel too.

'Depression is a common side effect of the illness,' I explained. 'I guess that's what comes from being divested of everything you have lived with and loved. And that's awful, but this disease takes things away from you – it takes away from who you are and the things you have always done. There are things I'm slightly scared about now – it's like being a child again and I just feel vulnerable, I think. And that's not me at all.'

But I didn't want the interview to be all doom and gloom. I felt a huge responsibility to try to show that I wasn't totally giving up just because I had Alzheimer's, because I didn't want others to give up if they had it too. Near the end I said: 'Thank God I'm otherwise fit and well, I suppose – it's just my brain that is a bit fucked.'

And we all laughed. Because, however bad things are, you've got to try to laugh.

After the interview a lovely photographer called Phil Coburn took pictures of me at home. Martin had arranged for me to have my hair and make-up done so I looked good in the snaps. We were both keen that people should see that I still looked bright and alert and I wasn't like the caricature of some little old lady with Alzheimer's.

The story broke in the *Mirror* on 4 July 2023. Within minutes of it dropping online, it had been shared on almost every news site you can imagine. The BBC and ITV both carried stories about it on the television news, and all the newspapers, including broadsheets like *The Times* and *The Daily Telegraph*, did big stories on me.

It was incredible how much people were affected by reading the stories about me and there were some wonderful messages too, both from colleagues from the world of TV and members of the public who had come to know me through my days on *GMTV* or through reading my *Mirror* column.

Lorraine Kelly called me a 'good, kind soul' and said: 'As expected, our much-loved Fiona is dealing with this shattering diagnosis with courage and optimism.'

Kate Garraway was so kind on *GMTV* and recalled a conversation we'd had recently on the phone. She said: 'The last conversation I had with her, which was only a few weeks ago, what she was doing was talking to me about Derek. Full of love for Derek, very close to Derek – and thinking about me dealing with Derek. Of course, I now think that she must have had in her mind that she would come to a place where Martin and her sons were going to be taking care of her.'

And Kate was right – I was thinking about that. About the pressure on an entire family when one member of that family becomes so unwell.

My old *Mirror* boss Piers Morgan tweeted: 'What incredibly sad news, but how typically honest & courageous of @realmissfiona to speak out about it. Lovely lady, wish her and her family all the best as they battle this horrible disease.'

Holly Willoughby called me 'brave' and Vanessa Feltz said I was 'incredible'.

I didn't feel either brave or incredible and it was quite overwhelming to hear all the lovely things people were saying about me. In the days that followed, strangers would come up to me in the street and ask how I was feeling. Even people who didn't want to come up and chat would nod at me and smile. Sometimes I didn't know why they were nodding and smiling and there were times when I entirely forgot that my story had been made public, but it was nice to feel support and love from people when I was out and about.

It made me feel secure.

29

Martin

Our main concern about going public with the news of Fiona's diagnosis was the impact it might have on the boys. Nat was then twenty-four and away a lot of time in the army. Mackenzie was twenty-one and still living at home. He was looking for a job but was also a huge help to me in looking after Fiona and making sure she had some company during the day. Fiona was adamant that she didn't ever want carers coming into our home, and she didn't need them at that point, but having Mackenzie there to keep an eye on things while I was at work put my mind at rest.

I asked the boys how they would feel if their mum's diagnosis came out in the media and they were relaxed about it all. They'd grown up with a mum who was frequently recognized in the street and who had been beamed into all their classmates' kitchens on breakfast TV, so it didn't worry them. They too thought it might be better if the stress of keeping a secret was lifted from all of us. Also, we all needed to be able to talk freely about what was happening at home.

The hospital had recommended to me support groups for

carers and family members, but with all due respect to the people who find those groups really valuable, the leaflets were all aimed at older people. The groups seemed to be catering for people who were retired and quite elderly; I just didn't feel they were for us. There didn't seem to be any support group – not that I'd really want a support group – for couples our age who were still working while going through this.

And Fiona didn't want to sit around for hours discussing her illness. We went for one session with a very lovely, but quite young, junior doctor. She was saying to Fiona: 'Tell me, how are you feeling?' and 'Can I explain how this might impact you and what the next stages might be?' But Fiona was very firm: 'Stop – I don't need this. I know everything about this disease because I've seen my mum and dad go through it and they're now ten feet under so I know what happens – I've lived with it for decades.'

We never went back for another of those sessions. And so, rightly or wrongly, we didn't discuss it much at all.

For years we had both always been so caught up with work that we didn't have a wide network of friends. Our families didn't live locally and we were quite insular. It meant we were coping with what was going on pretty much alone. I felt if Fiona could become more comfortable with the idea of people knowing about her illness then we both might be able to get some support through reaching out to the friends who we had until then kept out of the loop. They might pop over for a coffee and a chat with Fiona. Or it might lead to her meeting people in a similar situation, with early-onset Alzheimer's – people suffering like Fiona, who seemed invisible. Also, I knew at some point, if Fiona's condition worsened, we would need practical help and so more people would have to be told about the situation. I also carried a deep fear that one of the newspapers might find out about Fiona and come to us saying they were going to run the story. At that point we would have had no control over how we broke the news to our extended families and the wider world. Fiona had been such an independent and strong woman that it felt very important that she should tell her story on her terms and in her words. But she remained unconvinced for a long time and stubbornly refused to even discuss the prospect.

When Fiona was first diagnosed, I decided the two worst personality traits you could possibly have if you get Alzheimer's were being stubborn and being independent – and of course she was both. If she didn't want to take a drug or go for a test, she just wouldn't. And being independent is difficult too because, as time goes by, people with this illness have to become more reliant on others. For ages, Fiona refused – stubbornly – to accept this fact.

The reality was we couldn't stay hidden away for ever, barely going out or mixing with friends. But, if we did go out, I needed people to understand why Fiona's behaviour might seem different.

I'd only told my direct boss at work and the then-hosts of *This Morning*, Phillip Schofield and Holly Willoughby. I'd had to disappear for so many hospital appointments with Fiona that I felt I owed them an explanation as to what was going on.

They were all incredibly understanding and told me to take whatever time I needed to help my wife through this ordeal. But I hadn't told anyone else at all as I didn't want people gossiping about Fiona – she would hate that. It felt that level of secrecy was becoming unsustainable.

In the two months before the *Mirror* interview, we had a chance to tell Fiona's two brothers and her wider family about the diagnosis. David and Andrew were terribly upset, though I think they too had probably guessed something was changing. God knows they'd seen the signs before. But I don't think anyone who had seen Fiona in the months prior to the announcement would have found it a total shock when they heard the diagnosis – she was very good at masking her symptoms, but the forgetfulness and repeated conversations were becoming quite frequent.

The first interview where Fiona and I sat down with Alison and talked her through everything that had been happening over the past couple of years was almost a relief. There was no going back from that point and because there was someone else sitting at the table Fiona and I were able to discuss things that perhaps we wouldn't if there were just the two of us in the room.

Fiona was amazing during that interview, still so witty and sharp. When Alison turned to me and said, 'Martin, how did you feel when the consultant said it was Alzheimer's?', Fiona cut in laughing and said, 'Burdened!' And we all laughed. But then at other points in the interview, when we discussed how it was brain fog and anxiety that had first sent us to seek help from the menopause expert, Fiona had no recollection of that at all.

And we discussed how she had become more depressed since the diagnosis. Alison asked: 'Have you found yourself feeling low?'

'Not really,' replied Fiona.

I don't know if she was saying that because she was attempting to put on a brave face or whether she didn't remember how she had been feeling – or maybe it just didn't register with her that what she was feeling was depression. Maybe it was a combination of those things.

'Oh, but Fiona, you have,' I said.

'Really?' she replied, genuinely surprised. 'I don't think I've really been very depressed – well, I'm trying not to be.'

But in the next breath she admitted there were times when she woke up in the morning and thought, *Is it worth even getting up? I can't go to work and so I'll only end up going to the same old places for a coffee on my own or out for a walk.*

I knew the feeling that she couldn't work was weighing incredibly heavily upon Fiona and I desperately hoped for her sake, once the story was made public, there might be opportunities for her to perhaps make a documentary about living with Alzheimer's. Or there might be other offers of work. I was clinging to the thought that if she could get some work going again, she might feel a little less depressed and this in turn would help slow the illness. Because Fiona was still incredibly alert, articulate and sparky much of the time. She was able to remember key parts of her former life – looking after her parents or working with Eamonn Holmes on *GMTV* or the days when we met in LA, but the recent events and how she had become ill were lost to her.

I really didn't want the interview that came out publicly to be about me at all. I'm way more comfortable being out of the spotlight. And I didn't want people feeling sorry for me either. I wasn't the one who was having to suffer this terrible illness – it was Fiona, and I wanted the focus to remain on her.

So, when Alison asked how I was coping with supporting Fiona through it all, I answered honestly. 'It's what you sign up for when you become a couple,' I said. 'That when something like this comes along you have to get on and deal with it.'

I guess it was hardly the most romantic of answers, but it's what I believe.

'Well, I didn't bloody sign up for this either,' Fiona laughed.

I'm still not sure if she was talking about her illness or living with me!

I had no doubt that we were in this together and we were going to be dealing with whatever came next together. Alison asked Fiona if I'd really 'ramped it up' as a husband since this happened. Fiona was very kind and said I'd always been there for her, but I'm not sure that's entirely true.

'I don't think there's any doubt I have ramped it up,' I said. 'I have to think about things that I would never consider before. If I know I'm going out one evening, I have to consider what

Fiona is going to eat and make sure there is food in and ask Mackenzie to do the cooking. So yes, I do have to think about things in a way I never did before.'

We had such an open and honest chat that day about how we were both feeling about the changes that had hit our lives, but, while we were sitting there, I knew that by the next day Fiona would have forgotten the conversation, so what should I do then? Have the whole conversation again and again? Or did we just get on with life, day by day?

The story first broke online on 4 July and then in print the following morning. I was overwhelmed by the response. The story was covered on the BBC and ITV News, as well as in every national newspaper and website. It was a brilliant reminder of how loved Fiona was, but also of what a big issue Alzheimer's remains and how people were impacted by Fiona's story because they had lived with the illness in their families and knew the toll it takes. It was also a huge relief for me – the burden of secrecy was lifted and I felt bolstered by the support I received both from those closest to me and also from total strangers.

In the next few days, hundreds of articles were written about Alzheimer's, and particularly about early-onset Alzheimer's, which is devastating for younger people and their families. Once again I felt very proud of Fiona – she had got the whole country talking about an issue that mattered. She was still a brilliant journalist.

Two days after the story broke, Alison returned to interview Fiona for a follow-up piece about her reaction to the news.

'How do you feel about people knowing what you are going through?' Alison asked.

'Oh, I don't think anyone knows,' Fiona replied. 'I don't want to go around advertising what is happening.'

Even today, Fiona doesn't seem to acknowledge that people know she is unwell. She has done so much to raise awareness of this issue and yet now forgets she has done so. In one way that seems very sad, but in another, maybe that's just Fiona at her most fantastically independent and stubborn – still insisting she doesn't need people knowing her business, she doesn't need their help and definitely doesn't want their pity.

30

Fiona

We had a wonderful holiday in the late summer of 2023. Martin and I went to our little house in Italy for a fortnight and enjoyed the peace and quiet and being together. I don't like sitting in the direct sun of the day, but I was happy lazing in the shade of our garden, just watching the world go by. In the afternoons, he and I went for a drive and sat in a cafe and chatted.

Martin was still sticking needles in my stomach three times a day, but other than that we were able to forget all about this terrible illness. I didn't notice any particular difference from the drugs and that was worrying. I still wasn't my old self – I'd wake in the morning and feel strange, but then I wasn't sure how I would know if the treatment was working anyway.

When we got home from Italy we were back and forwards to the hospital every week or so. Martin would rush home around lunchtime, take me to the appointment, then go back to work.

After the holiday, I kept saying that I would like to be able to do some more television work. Martin spoke to a couple of production companies about whether they would be interested in me fronting a documentary about the impact of Alzheimer's on people and their families. I was also interested in travelling to the States, where some of the drug trials are more advanced. I'd hoped to meet people with Alzheimer's who had been trialling new drugs that had stabilized their condition or, in some cases, even reversed it.

I knew I could still read an autocue and make a documentary. I'd never felt fearful about live television and so filming a documentary didn't worry me at all. Well, that's what I said. And I wanted to do something useful. 'Maybe I'll organize an Alzheimer's convention,' I said to Martin one day. 'We'll all sit around and none of us will have a clue why we're there.' And we both laughed. We did still have a laugh together – but we had to. What was the alternative? To sit around crying about the future?

Everyone who Martin spoke to about the documentary project was more interested in a fly-on-the-wall style programme about me than something where I was out and about interviewing other sufferers or research scientists. And Martin and I have been in television long enough to know what they really wanted – to record on camera my worsening situation. Neither of us were keen on that; we didn't want to be followed by a film crew every time we went in for check-ups or test results, like some kind of boardroom scene from the BBC reality show, *The Apprentice*. And while a big part of me was desperate to get back to work, a lot of the time I was happy just getting up, going for a walk and then pottering around the house.

I felt vulnerable in strange situations – I was probably better off at home. But each morning I made an effort to get up, have a shower and put some nice clothes on. I was conscious that losing pride in your appearance was the start of things really going downhill. And for a while I did still see friends although I knew that often I would forget soon after I'd seen someone. Martin was very good at reminding me and would say things like, 'Oh, that was nice to see Amanda yesterday, wasn't it?' and I'd think, *Oh, was it? I'd forgotten I'd seen Amanda*. But it did help and jogged me to remember – or I thought I remembered.

But as time went by I lost some enthusiasm for going out and meeting people. I didn't want to talk about my illness and desperately tried to avoid it. I'd known from when my parents were ill that Alzheimer's can be the elephant in the room when people are together and chatting – now I was that elephant. As such, I preferred to stay at home and I never got bored – the hours just slipped past.

Martin would come home from work at about 7 p.m. and would cook for us both – he was obsessed about making sure I was getting a nutritious diet as by then I had totally lost interest in food and in cooking. But there was Martin, making sure I was getting plenty of iron and protein and whatnot. For years I'd taken great pride in cooking, but now I was happy picking at a takeaway or having nothing at all. I think it must have been connected to the illness – a part of that general sense of malaise that I had.

The boys were wonderful. Nat is like a big bear and he would come up and hug me and say: 'Love you, Mum.' And Mackenzie was amazing. He was still living at home, hoping to break into the fashion industry, and was such a support to me during the day when Martin was out at work.

Sometimes Martin and I would go for a drink at a local pub on a Friday evening. We'd chat about things that were going on and in many ways it was like nothing had changed. We didn't talk about my condition unless it would be me saying: 'When's my next appointment at the hospital?' because I was always forgetting when I had to go back there again.

We were in the pub one evening when all of a sudden there were hundreds of flashing blue lights, sirens wailing and a police helicopter hovering overhead. One of the inmates from Wandsworth Prison had escaped and was on the run.

'Oh, the poor thing, having to hide in alleyways in this weather,' I said.

'Oh, Fiona, you feel sorry for everyone,' Martin said.

'And what's wrong with that?' I demanded.

It was good that despite everything that had happened we were still able to have the same kind of 'lively' differences of opinion that we had always had. And thankfully they found the missing inmate, former British Army soldier Daniel Khalife, four days later.

That autumn of 2023, I had another big lift when *Woman & Home* magazine asked me to be the cover star for their January 2024 start-the-year issue. I was so chuffed they had chosen me.

When I went for the photo shoot and interview, they made

me feel so special. There were hair and make-up artists there and I posed in a series of outfits. The cover shot was me in a silver sequinned top with my hair styled and blowing backwards from a wind machine. In another shot I was wearing a blush-coloured mesh dress. And if I say so myself, I looked pretty good for a woman about to turn sixty-three!

In the interview they asked me about how I had been feeling since my diagnosis. I tried to be honest without depressing all their readers and I concluded the way I always did – with some hope. I said, 'I'm not about to give up. I know I can still have a great life. I'm just getting on with things. I'm pretending it hasn't happened and not giving it any space in my life at the moment. Or as little as I can. I've still got so much I want to do.'

Martin and I attended the Pride of Britain Awards that autumn again and had another wonderful evening. There were friends from television there, like Susanna Reid and lovely Ben Shephard, and there were so many others coming up to hug me and say hello. Some of them I knew, others I had no idea – I just made sure they all got a hug and the same big smile, so they'd have no idea which category they were in!

Similar things happened in the street too. Sometimes people would come up to me and say: 'Hi, Fiona, so lovely to see you,' and I wouldn't have a clue who they were. 'Oh, we met at such and such a place,' they'd say. I'd pretend to remember in order to keep them happy, but quite often I really didn't know. To be honest, that had been happening to me for years because when people see you on television they think they know you even when they don't – so it was perfectly possible these people didn't know me any more than I knew them!

By the start of 2024, I was feeling flatter again. I went out increasingly less and less often – I preferred being at home; it felt safer. Soon after, I developed the most horrible cystitis. It was awful – the sensation of needing to wee all the time seemed to overwhelm everything. I was tired of feeling unwell and just tired generally. With all of this, it became even harder writing this book and trying to get everything in the right order.

For the time being, I think I'll leave it to Martin to tell the story of how things progressed that year . . .

31

Martin

Towards the end of the drugs trial, Fiona was sick and tired of being injected three times a day. Who could blame her? But when the trial came to an end in the spring of 2024, we both lost the sense that we were fighting the advance of her illness.

We still didn't know whether Fiona was on the actual drug or a placebo, but I was convinced she was on the real thing because it felt as though the advance of her illness was being slowed. Fiona's condition plateaued for a year; then, when she stopped having the daily injections, she seemed to deteriorate quite quickly.

By that point, I was also more realistic about what chance there actually was of any drug becoming available in time to make a big difference for Fiona. The drug she was trialling was being made in the UK so, if it got the go-ahead for use on the NHS, it was possible that it could be available within a year or so. But I also knew that NICE had blocked the rollout of some drugs, saying the enormous cost couldn't be justified against the little additional time it was giving people with Alzheimer's. Gradually – and it did take a while – I had to come to terms with the reality that any drug would be too late to make a difference and there was nothing I could do about it.

The trial ending had a psychological impact on Fiona too. While it was ongoing, we had hospital appointments every four or five weeks and I was giving her the injections three times a day, so she probably felt she was in a process that might make her better. But, once that was over, there was no process, no hospital appointments that might reveal new hope, nothing. I wonder if she felt she had nothing left to cling to and, as a result, her condition went downhill.

I kept in touch with the head of the trials programme in case there were any other drugs they were working on which Fiona might be eligible to test, but there was nothing immediately suitable. And, as her condition deteriorated, there were fewer suitable drugs being trialled. I kept trying but, without that lifeline, all we could do was wait to see how slowly – or quickly – Fiona's illness would advance.

As 2024 progressed, all the things we enjoyed doing together – eating good food, drinking nice wine, going to lovely places, travelling – started to become too difficult for her. Of course we'd had to make adjustments – I'd increasingly have to talk Fiona through the different choices on a menu if we went out for dinner. Or when we went on holiday, I'd do the packing to make sure she didn't forget anything. And then I'd have to be careful she didn't get anxious or confused at the airport. But, up to this point, she still wanted to go out and would enjoy a glass of wine and a gossip. And she loved going to Italy and lying by the pool.

There were still moments when we would laugh together and I'd see a spark of the old Fiona. There was one day when I had invited the dementia choir set up by the actress Vicky McClure onto *This Morning*. I spent ages building up to suggesting to Fiona that she might like to join the choir or something similar. One evening, I came home from work and said as casually as I could: 'Oh, we had Vicky McClure from *Line of Duty* on the show today and she has got this amazing choir for people who have dementia and, er, I was thinking . . .'

'Can you just stop right there?' Fiona interrupted.

'It's just a choir,' I said, despite realizing the battle was already lost. 'It's really good for people to share and get together and er, have a nice time . . .'

'You can take your choir and fuck right off!' Fiona replied, laughing. 'And you can take your jigsaws with you too.'

So that's what Fiona thought about singing and the jigsaw puzzle I'd bought her for Christmas. She was still too sharp to think that all the activities that people with Alzheimer's are supposed to try were actually going to make a blind bit of difference in the face of the enormous thing that was coming for her.

Since Fiona's diagnosis, we had done lots of stories on *This Morning* about dementia; each time we were inundated with people ringing in to share their experiences. From this, I realized how many families were feeling very forgotten about and were having to cope with the most awful situations entirely alone. Our personal situation wasn't as bad as some of those shared by viewers but, despite the fun moments when we could still laugh at silly things at home, we could see that Fiona was losing enthusiasm for what was going on around her. As the weeks went by, she barely left the house.

By the summer of 2024, we had adjusted to a new routine. On a normal day, I would wake at seven and go downstairs to make a coffee. If Fiona heard me, she might come down too. I was in control of all her medication to ensure she took the correct amounts, so I would give her an antidepressant tablet and make her a cup of tea, then get myself ready for work.

Fiona would often say to me: 'What shall I do now?'

'Why don't you go back to bed for a couple of hours?' I'd say. 'It's still early.'

'Where do I go to bed?' she would ask.

'In the bedroom,' I'd reply and point her back to the staircase in her own home. It had reached the point where she no longer knew where her bedroom was.

Sometimes when I woke up she might already be dressed, because she had got up in the middle of the night and put clothes on. During the late spring and early summer, it would get light at 4 a.m. and she'd be very disorientated, not knowing if it was day or night and therefore getting up at all hours.

We would have this discussion and then I would go to work and Fiona would go back to sleep until she heard Mackenzie up and about. He would make her some breakfast, but she rarely ate much, then he would suggest she could do something or they might go for a walk, but usually Fiona preferred just to sit and look out of the window.

Sometimes a friend might call to see if she wanted to meet up, but she would either say no or more likely not answer the call. If a friend was coming over, I would have to prepare Fiona for the visit so she wasn't confused when they arrived. It was becoming harder and harder for her to remember people and places. She was also becoming confused by text messages and unable to remember who had sent them to her and why. She gave up reading or sending emails or looking at magazines, so she didn't really do very much. That was the pattern day after day – not much happened – and Fiona didn't want anything to happen.

I would nip out of work to buy food and get any prescriptions Fiona needed. And then, when I got home at about seven, I'd set about making dinner.

Fiona had developed a fascination with apples and could eat four apples while I was cooking. I was just relieved that her appetite seemed to be returning. When I googled 'apples and Alzheimer's', it said they can be great for people with the illness. She'd also eat a big fresh kefir yoghurt, which is a probiotic and good for the gut. She stopped drinking alcohol because of the pain she was feeling from what we believed to be cystitis and because she just didn't fancy it – she was happy drinking coconut water. After we ate dinner, I might read or check my work emails and Fiona would sit next to me. When I got in from work, it seemed she would rarely leave my side.

We might watch television for a bit, but Fiona wasn't able to engage with what was happening – I think often it was just bright colour on a screen to her. Sometimes she would focus and have a reaction; for instance, we might watch *MasterChef* and she would recognize a contestant from a previous round and say, 'I've seen this before.'

Every evening she would ask, 'How did your show go today?' I'd talk about what happened, but then literally sixty seconds later she would say again: 'How did the show go today?' And again I would explain how it went.

By the fifth time she had asked exactly the same question, I'd just say 'fine'. I tried so hard to remain patient, but it was difficult. And I'm only human. Anyone who thinks they could endlessly explain the same thing over and over again without ever becoming frustrated or losing their patience just needs to try it. Not once, not now and again, but every single day.

I had suggested we could get a carer to come in and be with Fiona during the day, but she absolutely refused. So then I suggested a 'housekeeper', thinking that it was the word 'carer' she objected to. But the mere suggestion of 'housekeeper' was like a red flag to Fiona. I could see her thinking, *Hmm, that sounds a bit like a carer to me and I'm not having that.* So she could be incredibly switched on when she chose to be and she had a defence mechanism that meant that while she knew on one level that she had Alzheimer's, on another she wouldn't accept it and refused to let anybody else say or do anything that would indicate she did. But I knew at some point somehow I would have to insist she had someone with her during the day for company and to give her some interaction when I wasn't around – the challenge was how could I make her agree to it?

Our conversations were often rooted in the past. She would

talk frequently about when she was working with Eamonn Holmes on *GMTV* or when her parents were ill and she was travelling back and forth to visit them. Otherwise the things we talked about were very much in the present. Things like 'Shall we watch television?' or 'How was work?' or 'Do you want a drink?' Occasionally she picked up things she might have heard on the radio news such as 'What's all this with Huw Edwards?' So she knew exactly who the lead presenter of *BBC News at Ten* was and understood he was involved in a story that was quite big, but she wasn't aware of why he was being talked about. I would tell her what the Huw Edwards story was and she would say, 'Oh gosh, that's awful,' but two minutes later it was gone again.

Fiona's specialist explained to me that her long-term memory was functioning better than the short-term so yes, she could remember who Huw Edwards was and yes, she was aware that he was involved in some kind of scandal because it was on the news. But what was missing was the ability to retain the recent memory of the cause of the scandal and that was what she had to keep being reminded of.

It was like that with a lot of the news stories that came and went. If we were in the car and music came on the radio, she would frequently be able to remember the name of the song and the band who performed it, when I hadn't got a clue, but she wouldn't be able to follow the plot of a TV drama or the conversation on a chat show.

At weekends we might go for a drive together or I could sometimes persuade her to go for a walk. 'Which season is it?'

she would ask as we were strolling across the Common. The buds might be on the trees in the early days of spring, but Fiona felt lost in time.

Often she felt quite depressed – the antidepressants didn't seem to be helping at all – and so after a while we abandoned them completely. It didn't seem to make the slightest difference. The doctors said getting her outside in the fresh air would be good for her, but it was such a struggle to persuade her to leave the house and if she didn't want to go out, what was I supposed to do? Manhandle her out of the front door?

I was busy with work at that time. We'd had big changes at *This Morning* with Phillip Schofield leaving, Holly Willoughby stepping down after the pressures of a serious kidnap threat, and Cat Deeley and Ben Shephard becoming the new hosts in March 2024. It meant there was a lot to sort out to make the show the best it possibly could be, but being that busy actually helped me. I loved going into work – not because it was an escape from what was going on at home, but because it gave me structure and normality. And it meant that I didn't have time to think about what was to come for Fiona.

For both of us.

Around this time, Fiona had been complaining of cystitis or a urinary tract infection (UTI), which can be very common for women – and men – and causes a horrible feeling that you need to urinate all the time. When you do wee, there is a burning pain.

At first I bought some powder for cystitis over the counter at the local pharmacy, but Fiona said it did nothing to ease the problem. Then we were back and forth with the doctor, who put Fiona on antibiotics. When they didn't work, even stronger antibiotics were prescribed. Still her condition didn't improve and the pain was causing her real distress. She even went for an MRI scan to see if it could identify the cause of the problem, but it remained a mystery.

The doctors said there was no evidence Fiona even had a UTI, although it was possible she might have had one a couple of months previously. Yet, for whatever reason, her mind was telling her she was still in pain. It was so difficult because she was constantly complaining of this pain, but there was nothing we could do to ease it for her.

The pain began to dominate her life and meant she was reluctant to leave the house, even with me. If a friend was coming to visit, she would say that the pain was too much and she would ask them to come another day. For months and months, the first thing she would say to me when I stepped in the door from work was, 'Oh, I've got such awful cystitis.'

It was like clockwork. 'I'm still in such pain,' she would say. 'When is this going to go away, do you think?' Then she would repeat that over and over again until she went to sleep.

Because we always had so many appointments coming up, all I could keep saying was: 'Well, hopefully the next time we go back to the doctor they'll be able to tell us what it is and we'll get it sorted out.' Of course a few minutes later, she would ask the same question again and all I could do was give the same answer. But then if Mackenzie came in or Nat was at home and one of them walked into the room, Fiona would say,

'Oh, hi! How are you? What have you been up to today?' She'd be bright and cheerful and there would be no mention of cystitis at all. And it made me wonder what was behind it all.

As I've said, the thought of going out or a visitor coming over to the house instantly led to her complaining of the pain. There's no doubt she seemed to be in huge discomfort, but I also wondered if it was connected to an anxiety about having to do things that scared or overwhelmed her. Or whether the thought of pain came and went depending on what was happening.

We went backwards and forwards, and backwards and forwards, to the doctors, consultants, specialists. You name it, we saw them. Fiona had every test, every scan, ultrasound and blood test going, but still no one could work out what the problem was. Also, we couldn't tell if the Alzheimer's was in some way connected. Certainly, the growing sense of confusion that Fiona was struggling with made it hard for her to explain exactly what she was going through – we were desperate to find a way to alleviate the pain and distress that she was enduring. Often she would cry because everything was so overwhelming.

It is hard to see someone who was as independent and confident as Fiona become as vulnerable as she now is. I think she feels safest when I'm around. She does something that experts call 'shadowing'. It's when someone with the disease follows their partner or carer everywhere they go to be close to them. This gives them a greater sense of security when they feel very lost and disorientated by things going on around them. At the same time, they can be difficult or unreasonable with the person closest to them, while with everyone else they can be absolutely fine.

Fiona can still make an effort to put on a bright face for some people if they pop over to visit, but with me, if there's something she doesn't want to do, like get in the car for a hospital appointment, she will totally withdraw. Particularly when she was struggling with pain in the autumn of 2024, it felt like other people were getting the best of Fiona while I had to deal with her when she was snappy or refusing to do anything I suggested or was crying and utterly desolate. But there was no point in my getting frustrated. Even if we had that conversation about how she was behaving or how low she was feeling, she would have forgotten about it by the next day anyway – talking things through didn't help.

It was difficult to know whether Fiona's increasing confusion might have been caused by the pain she was experiencing. And what no one could tell us was whether her condition would return to how she had been at the end of the trials if they managed to reduce the pain. Would that make her more alert? Or would she stabilize where she was, at that point where she couldn't remember where the bedroom was? No one seemed to know.

In the summer of 2024, I had hoped that a trip to Italy might distract Fiona from the pain she was constantly complaining about. We flew out with Mackenzie and had arranged for friends to come and join us there. But the whole trip was a disaster. From the moment we arrived, Fiona was crying and in a terrible state of distress. It was a mixture of horrible physical pain and the worst of her anxiety. It was clear that she was desperate to go home and she wouldn't feel better until she was back there. I didn't know what to do as our friends were arriving to join us, but the thought of that was only making Fiona worse.

In the end, I had to book the first flights back I could find. The holiday lasted less than seventy-two hours, but once Fiona was on the plane home she started to feel better. The next day I got her an emergency appointment with a specialist, but he struggled to work out what was causing the problem.

Fiona was clearly much happier back home and less anxious. I still tried to plan things for us to do at weekends as I felt it was important for Fiona to get out of the house whenever she could be persuaded, but it was so difficult.

One weekend I said, 'Let's go down to the coast.' I had a part share in a boat down on the South Coast – I hoped Fiona might enjoy the fresh air down there and feel more relaxed away from London.

Nat and his girlfriend were coming too. We managed to get Fiona, crying, out of the house and into the car. Nat was desperately trying to encourage her. 'Come on, Mum,' he said. 'It's like being in the army, you have to do things you don't want to do, but it'll be worth it.'

Fiona was insistent she didn't want to go, but I really thought she would enjoy it once we got there. We drove for about half an hour but the traffic was so terrible, we barely went any distance. Meanwhile, Fiona was still crying and saying to Nat's girlfriend over and over again about how she was in terrible pain.

The whole thing was a complete and utter disaster.

I can't do this, I thought, and swung the car around.

'Don't worry, Fiona,' I said. 'We're going home.'

She changed in an instant. Now she was smiling and laughing. It was so frustrating as I couldn't work out if there was a physical cause of the pain or if her mind was conjuring it when she was in situations in which she felt uncomfortable. Either way, it was incredibly distressing for her and upsetting for the entire family.

As the autumn of 2024 progressed, her condition deteriorated further and she spent a lot of time in bed, either in pain or sleeping. The problems Fiona was struggling with also impacted her bowel habits. I don't like to talk about it as I desperately want to keep her dignity intact, but at the same time I think it's important that people understand how terrible this disease can be for those who have it – and those who love them and have to care for them. No one can prepare you for what it's like, having to help your wife when she's sobbing over the indignity this disease has wrought upon her. It's the worst possible thing.

Finally, towards the end of 2024, we found a specialist who was able to work out what the issue was. He recommended an operation to repair the problem. I don't want to go into all the awful details of what Fiona had been suffering, but her pain was very real and only an operation could make things better. I was concerned about the impact of Fiona undergoing an anaesthetic and surgery when she was already so disorientated, but the boys and I were just desperate to do anything that might alleviate her suffering. For the six weeks before the operation, Fiona was doubled up in agony. It was devastating to see her like that. All I could tell her was that she was booked in for an operation and she would be getting better soon.

Christmas Day was tough. In the past, we would have gone down to Dorset with the boys or gone out for dinner – it was always a lovely, fun day. I did think about booking a restaurant so the boys would have a nice time, but I knew Fiona was in pain and I was worried that if we got there and then she couldn't eat her meal, we would have to leave it all and rush home. So instead I bought food and tried to do Christmas dinner as best I could at home.

Fiona was all right for about half an hour or forty minutes, but then she just had to go to bed because she was feeling so ill and her mood was so low. It wasn't much of a Christmas for the boys.

It's tough for them. They see their mum like this and it's very upsetting, but what choice do we have but to keep on going? I do encourage them to go out with their friends, and Nat spends time with his girlfriend, because I think it's important that they get a break from what's happening at home – I don't want them to be psychologically damaged by this. We have a close relationship and talk a lot about Fiona and how she is feeling, but it is difficult to discuss the impact it has had on us. I think we all feel that whatever we are going through, it's nothing compared with what Fiona is enduring, so we just get on with what needs to be done.

In those final days of 2024, Fiona was barely eating and the painkillers weren't even touching the sides. This was a woman who'd had the highest pain threshold I have ever known, but of course we didn't know if Alzheimer's was impacting the feelings of pain and it was impossible for her to explain that to us.

'Please help me!' she begged me several times.

I felt utterly helpless – it seemed there was nothing I could do.

'We could go to A&E?' I suggested a couple of times when it was really bad.

'No, no, I can't go there,' she replied.

She was too scared to leave the house and I was terrified we would turn up at the hospital and have to wait twelve hours in a corridor just to be handed more of the same painkillers we already had. And then when I did say, 'Right, that's it, I'm calling 999,' Fiona seemed to improve, so I had no idea what was really going on. All we could do was wait for the operation and hope it ended the physical pain, which might then impact the mental anxiety it was causing too.

'But what if they can never sort this out?' Fiona said, crying.

'They will, they will,' was all I could say.

The pain often made her confusion worse to the point of borderline delirium, a condition that can happen to people with Alzheimer's when they become rapidly unsettled in the space of a few hours. One weekend, Nat was home from the army and making tea in the kitchen while Fiona and I sat watching television and she was in that borderline state.

She became terribly distressed. 'Who's that man in the kitchen?' she asked me.

'That's Nat,' I said gently. 'Our son. He's home for the weekend.'

She was in such a state that she didn't even seem upset that she had asked the question. Fortunately, Nat didn't hear or I think he would have been devastated.

The operation was booked in for 6 January 2025. Fiona was in a terrible way the night before. It was the same evening that *Dancing on Ice* started on ITV, which Holly Willoughby hosts. I had worked with Holly for years and we are good friends as well as colleagues, but that evening was a stark reminder of how our lives had gone in such different directions.

I watched the start of the programme and Holly was there wearing a fabulous gown, smiling and looking amazing. Then there was me trying to look after Fiona, who was feeling really unwell. I spent the rest of the show caring for my wife, who was crying in the bathroom, utterly desolate. I couldn't help but think how my life and Holly's had diverged so much in the space of a year.

But that's the roll of the dice.

The next morning, we had to be at the hospital for 6.30 a.m. Just getting Fiona into the taxi was incredibly difficult. She was crying, doubled up in pain, and really didn't want to leave the house. I think she kind of knew we were going to hospital for the surgery but didn't really understand why, and however many times I would say this was going to make her better, moments later she would have forgotten again.

Fiona went down to the operating theatre at about 9 a.m. and was there for four hours. When the consultant came out, he said he'd been able to repair the problem and had also found a cyst wrapped around her bowel, which he'd removed.

'I can understand why she was in such terrible pain,' he said to me. 'Hopefully now she will start to get better.'

But Fiona's recovery would prove tough. Again, she had a case of delirium probably caused by the general anaesthetic and her body recovering from the operation in addition to Alzheimer's. She didn't know where she was; she thought the doctors and nurses were scammers dressed up in uniforms and at one point she didn't know who Nat was when he came to visit.

The boys and I were allowed to take it in turns to be at her bedside twenty-four hours of the day because she was so confused. Nat was with Fiona in the early hours of one morning when she woke and was insistent she was leaving – 'Get out of my way, I'm going home!' she was shouting at him. She was still wired up to machines, but was trying to pull the cables off herself. Nat was attempting everything to calm her down, but she was in too much of a state. I slept through him calling me, so he had to come home in a cab to fetch me. By the time I dashed back there, she had calmed down completely and was happily walking up and down the ward.

A couple of days later, Fiona was allowed home. We could only hope that now, back home, safe and secure, her confusion might ease a little.

32

January 2025

As I start writing this chapter in 2025, Fiona needs a lot of help. She needs help showering and brushing her teeth. She can do these things physically, but is unable now to think about how she should do them. I wash Fiona's hair because she wouldn't know what shampoo or conditioner to use or how wet her hair needs to be or that she must rinse the soap suds out afterwards. And most nights I'll say, 'Right, we need to brush our teeth before we go to bed,' and I'll put the tooth-paste on the brush and hand it to her. She is still very stubborn and doesn't like brushing her teeth or feeling that she is being told what to do, so she rails against it. But this has to be the way, because the worst thing that could happen, after having got her through the pain of last year, would be for her to get some kind of tooth infection when she is vulnerable.

She can put clothes on, but may not put them on the right way around, so she does need help dressing. I try to lay out clothes for her to put on in the morning, but she tends to get attached to particular items of clothing and will wear them over and over again. For example, she may start sleeping in a jumper that she particularly likes until I'm able to get it away from her and put it in the washing machine.

She can no longer use her phone; she will look at it but isn't able to work out sending a text message and doesn't even think to do that. There have also been things I've had to do for her that are far worse than putting toothpaste on her brush. I'd ask myself: *Can this get any worse, can this really get any worse?*

But then it does. And that becomes routine. I'll think to myself: *Well, I don't want anyone else to have to do this for Fiona, so there's no option but to keep going.* I'm just trying to give her the best care I can and to make her feel as safe and secure as possible. And Fiona wants me to do that personal care for her – she trusts me. I have seen her at her lowest ebb, but at least it's me there with her. I know it's not her anyway – it's an illness doing this to her and that's what I say to her: *This isn't you, Fiona, it's the illness.*

Being brutally honest, I wish Fiona had contracted cancer. Maybe she will – wouldn't that just take the biscuit?! It's a shocking thing to say, but at least then she might have had a chance of a cure, and certainly would have had a treatment pathway and an array of support and care packages. But that's not there for Alzheimer's. Just like there are no funny or inspiring TikTok videos or fashion shoots with smiling, healthy, in-remission survivors. After someone is diagnosed with Alzheimer's, they are pretty much left to their own devices. There is nothing more that can be done and you are left to cope alone. Bit by bit, it takes everything. Through time, even the most glamorous, glittering star – such as Fiona was – will be wiped away. Alzheimer's steals looks along with dissolving memory. Sometimes Fiona has the unmistakable 'dementia eyes' when she stares blankly ahead. This isn't always, but when it does happen it is accompanied by a sense of fear and deep confusion.

Across Britain there are dedicated hospitals and centres of excellence for cancer, heart disease and even eye conditions. There is nothing like that for dementia and Alzheimer's – even though it is now the country's biggest killer. It was first given a name with a diagnosis in 1915 – that's 110 years ago – and I would argue it is no closer to being cured today. Or, even more shockingly, no closer to being cared for.

I don't have it in me to become a poster boy for Alzheimer's campaigns. I have a wife who is slipping away from us day by day and we have altered our lives to cope with this heartbreaking condition. But our whole existence, especially for our children, has been wrecked so much already that we will use this book to raise awareness and then do no more. I refuse to let the disease claim more of our misery – it's supped enough on our grief.

There will be no marathons from me, no fundraising dinners, no 'why me?' or 'why us?' articles. We will have done our bit and, to be honest, I'm not sure even mass fundraising campaigns would secure the holy grail of a cure for dementia. Perhaps we just have to accept that the brain is the most complex organ known to mankind – smarter than the smartest AI software –

with billions of nerve cells that control emotions, movement and thoughts, and we will never fully understand why it shuts down prematurely (because dementia is a disease and not simply a result of old age). Would money be better spent on proper care and pathways to support the families of those affected and to allow victims a chance to gradually disappear with dignity or even, in a few cases, to live well for a bit?

From my day job as the editor of the UK's most famous morning show, I admit for many years I shied away from discussing Alzheimer's as a topic among the 2,000-plus items we covered each season. It wasn't until Fiona's diagnosis that we took up the cudgels.

When I first mentioned Fiona's diagnosis to my *This Morning* colleagues Phillip Schofield and Holly Willoughby, they were supportive and kind. Holly always went out of her way to ask about Fiona whenever we were alone. She genuinely cared and I will always be grateful for her kind words, which cheered me when little else could. I haven't spoken previously about the difficult times we went through as a family during the Schofield scandal in the early summer of 2022, but perhaps I should briefly. It was bemusing to see film crews, reporters and even a satellite truck outside my house for eight days straight when the story broke, but it was not wonderful to have my wife chased down the street by the paparazzi as she went out for a coffee. Some of the film crews had worked with me during my years as a reporter on risky foreign shoots in warzones, yet here they were in leafy Wandsworth, apologizing for their newsdesk's appetite for doorstepping a backroom boy. I'd probably have done the same if I'd been the editor.

It's three years on, but now I finally know what friends meant when they asked me after the diagnosis: 'But are *you* OK?' My response at that time – and for months afterwards – was: 'Yes, of course I'm fine.' It wasn't me who had been given the death sentence and all I felt was sympathy for my wife. But, as time has passed, I came to understand that if I were to fall ill or worse, the whole house of cards would collapse. I have had to stay well for Fiona. Sorting the bank accounts, utility direct debits, hospital appointments, clothes, washing, parking permits, shopping, cooking, tidying the house – in fact, all the stuff I took for granted because Fiona dealt with it (as well as her own career) – became my responsibilities, along with a seven-day-a-week job. It was knackering. There were times I felt drained, physically and emotionally. On top of the stress, the boys and I are enduring a kind of living grief – a slow goodbye to the woman we love.

Just before Christmas 2024, I decided we had to get some additional help with caring. Mackenzie was taking on a lot of the responsibility for looking after Fiona when I was at work, but I didn't want him to become his mum's full-time carer at twenty-three – we desperately needed a bit of support.

Because Fiona had insisted she didn't want or need a carer, I said that I had decided to employ a housekeeper to help us keep on top of the washing and cleaning. In reality, the lady who came to work for us was a trained carer, but I couldn't tell

Fiona that as she would have been appalled. Gradually, though, she took on more and more caring duties and Fiona didn't object, even though she would never accept that she was in the house to help care for her.

Fiona tends to sleep longer each morning now. A year or so ago, she would get up at seven when I went to work, but she doesn't do that now – she has her own room and sleeps through until mid-morning. When she gets up, she will come downstairs and see who is in the house, which will be either her carer or Mackenzie. They will make her something to eat and drink as she is no longer able to work out how to do that.

If Fiona is in the kitchen, it wouldn't occur to her to make a cup of coffee. She doesn't know where the mugs and coffee are kept and she wouldn't be able to work out how to turn on the kettle any more. I don't really worry about her being unsafe in the kitchen now as she would never think to use the appliances or the oven. Those are just some of the many things that are now outside the range of what she understands.

For the rest of the day, Fiona will just sit quietly or she may do something like move things around her room. She can stand and look at an item of clothing for a long time, trying to work out what it is, or she'll forget what she's doing and wander into a different room.

I'm hoping that as she recovers from the operation and starts to feel a bit better, she might agree to go for a walk more often with Mackenzie or me, though she still wouldn't do that with her carer as she would be very conscious that she was being 'taken for a walk'. At the moment, she still thinks of the carer as a housekeeper, so why would they be going out for a walk together?

In the evenings, I cook and then we sit and watch television together for a while. Even after the operation, Fiona frequently thinks she needs to go to the toilet even when she doesn't, which I think must be an anxiety issue. If we're sitting on the sofa, she will get up and say she needs the bathroom, but then she can't remember where it is or where the stairs are – I have to guide her to the staircase in her own home.

Fiona rarely leaves the house now. I use a variety of excuses to get myself outside for respite. The most common white lie is 'I'm shopping for our dinner', which is often true as I cook all our meals, but it also means a snatched hour in our local cafe where I can feel part of the real world.

There have been a couple more episodes of extreme confusion. She talks about the pain again and has had what almost seems like a panic attack. One night she became incredibly distressed: 'I just want my mum and dad,' she kept saying.

'Oh, Fiona, your mum and dad haven't been with us for many years,' I replied. But that just made her more agitated.

'You're lying,' she shouted. 'Get me my husband!'

All I could do was to keep trying to calm her down – 'Fiona, I am your husband,' I said.

'No, you are not,' she insisted.

The experts say you are not supposed to challenge someone with Alzheimer's when they're saying things that are completely wrong, but it's very difficult when you are in that moment and you are just desperately hoping you might be able to get through to them. What am I supposed to say when she says: 'You're not my husband!'? Some men might find that painful – and obviously it's not nice – but I don't feel hurt by it because I know that isn't Fiona talking: it's the illness that has taken her mind.

It feels as though I have read a million books and online articles about how best to cope with a partner with Alzheimer's. Some of the advice I agree with – but other bits I'm not so sure about. I think you just have to trust your instinct and deal with whatever is thrown at you as best you can in that moment. By trying to live up to being the perfect Alzheimer's partner, you are just heaping even more pressure on yourself when there is already so much.

And every day is different. The morning after Fiona told me, 'You're not my husband,' she was totally calm and far less confused and we were able to have a conversation. They are limited conversations now, but they are still possible. Fiona lives in the present and just comments on what she sees going on around her. She doesn't have a future – I mean she can't think about or imagine a future. And she doesn't have an immediate past – anything from thirty seconds ago or five minutes ago. So really it's just existing: she is existing in the present. Her brain almost seems to choose when it wishes to be quite lucid and when it just wants to become vacant, but I'm sure everyone with Alzheimer's is different, so there is no linear path to be followed.

When we are together, I feel I have to constantly be talking and keeping her spirits up to avoid a silence when she might start repeating, 'Oh, I feel awful, this is so awful!' I'll talk about anything and everything to distract her mind from the situation she's in. And I too repeat stories and anecdotes that I think she will like because, if she's forgotten them, what does it matter? It prevents her from thinking about Alzheimer's for a short while and the darkness she lives in. But it's tiring. Exhausting. And some evenings, if Fiona is complaining, I'll say, 'Oh, maybe you should go to bed.' Then I hate myself for saying that and for suggesting that she leave me alone. But it's the only relief I might get from the constant repetition of 'I feel awful' and 'Please help me'. However many times I try to reassure her, she has forgotten that reassurance moments later, so I have to do it over and over again. There's no escape.

We rarely go out. There's no doubt that some people we used to know don't get in touch as often. The dinner-party invitations have dried up and it can feel isolating. It's not that Fiona would even want to go out for dinner but sometimes it would be nice to be asked. I don't think people are deliberately trying to exclude us, they're just not sure what to say and so they say nothing at all.

And it does feel lonely. It feels selfish to say that because this is not about me – it's about Fiona and she's the one who is really suffering in all this. She's the one who feels lonely and scared and is often in pain. Sometimes when I'm going out she will say, 'Please don't leave me,' because she wants me to be close by. And it breaks my heart that my strong, independent wife has become so vulnerable.

I have become quieter and more introverted myself. I don't really have close friends I can talk to because, as I said earlier, for years my life revolved around work and Fiona. The boys are a big support to me, and people at work have been very kind, but what can anyone say? They stopped asking 'Did you have a nice weekend?' They know what my weekends are like. They don't want to bring it up because they know I want to get away from the awfulness of home when I'm at work.

Their motives are good, but still, bit by bit, I have become excluded from social conversations. I am not part of a world where weekends and Christmases are about fun and partying and laughing – that's not our world now.

At the time of writing, I have just finished my almost-ten-year stint as editor at *This Morning*. I'm proud of what I achieved – the longest tenure of any boss and seven consecutive National Television Awards during my run – but it was time to go. I feel I still have more to give in that world, but it became impossible to work the schedule I imposed on myself and be the principal responsible adult for someone with Alzheimer's. I could manage three or four days perhaps, but not the full-on white heat of running what many see as a national institution. The day we announced I was leaving the show, it was the front-page lead in *The Sun* – and I'm not even on screen! That unhealthy fascination the newspapers seem to have about the goings-on on *This Morning* meant my weekends were often taken up refuting stories or dealing with issues on a phone that always had to be on – so something had to give.

I made it clear to friends and colleagues that while I was

sorting out a better work–life balance and stepping back from that particular front line, I was not about to become the Mother Teresa of Wandsworth. I want to continue working and am setting up a small podcast project that I hope might become big. What I really want is distraction from all that is going on – and interesting conversation, which I'm lacking more and more in our isolated lives.

It's a wretched situation that's not going to get better. Day by day, in front of our eyes, we watch the illness slowly advance.

I know I need to stay well for the sake of the whole family, but looking after myself is difficult when I'm spending so much time caring for my wife. And the only other time I have left is spent working and doing the things that make me feel like there are some elements of my life that are still normal. It's hard – and this could go on for years.

I did have one weekend alone in Italy after Fiona had the operation as I had to sort out some problems with our house. At first I thought: *Oh, it'll be great to get a bit of time and space on my own.* I knew Fiona was being well looked after by her carer and the boys, plus people kept telling me I needed a break. But it was just me on my own in the middle of winter in Italy. And, without Fiona, it wasn't the same. I was lonely and quite quickly I just felt guilty in case she was wondering where I was, and I was constantly stressed in case she was upset about me not being there. There's no respite in this situation, wherever I am. Even writing that makes me feel bad, as again the person really suffering in all this is Fiona – this is about her.

I now think the term 'Alzheimer's' is just too broad – the differences in the way it impacts people are too enormous to be covered by one word. Some people with the illness may be able to play concert-standard piano, but others are struggling to speak. There has to be a better way of defining it so the differences in different people's conditions are better understood.

Now, when I meet people I haven't seen for a while, they will ask how Fiona is getting on, but I don't give too much detail. Sometimes they might tell me supposedly inspiring stories about people with Alzheimer's who are happily doing jigsaws or gardening each day. And I know it helps some people to cling to such stories, but that's not the Alzheimer's my wife has – she is depressed and anxious and sad.

And, because I've googled her illness and what her future might be like, my algorithms keep sending me ads about old-age care homes. But I don't want to be spending our time with people twenty or thirty years older than us. Fiona may have this illness, but she doesn't want that either – she remains very conscious of not wanting to be treated like she's old or sick, so we just carry on at home doing the best we can.

I'm lucky because I have two great kids and I can afford some help, but many people have to cope entirely on their own with a partner who has Alzheimer's – and I don't know how they manage that. There are people who have to give up their jobs to care for a loved one, living off their pension or from whatever they can scrape together.

In my darkest moments, I have thought about what the

future might hold. Do we reach a point where I have to say, 'OK, we can't cope here,' because Fiona wouldn't want me and the kids to do the really basic stuff that is so undignified? Will she have to go into a care home? But it all feels wrong – we are still relatively young. How could Fiona move into a care home meant for old people with walking frames? At this stage of our life, it feels so, so wrong.

There's no question of us being anywhere near that yet – we want Fiona at home with us. Besides, she is still able to make such decisions for herself. But I can't help looking into the future and thinking that there will be a time when she isn't able to make those decisions and the responsibility will fall on me. What will I do then, when I have to decide how she can best be cared for? How will I cope, knowing what this would have once meant to my fiercely independent wife?

I'd like to tell you Fiona is content in the situation into which she has been forced. I'd like to give readers some sense that she is at peace. But that wouldn't be the truth. She isn't – she is frustrated every single day. And depressed. In some ways, she has an active brain. She constantly says she wants to work, but she knows deep down that she can't. She knows she cannot hold a conversation and she forgets what she wants to tell people. I can see her searching for the thread of a conversation, but then it's gone and that's incredibly hard. At that point, she will give up and crumple. She tries to fight it, but it's too hard.

Fiona's latest fixation, coming from her clogged-up brain, is a suspicion that we have kidnapped her and won't let her go home to her mum and dad. Again, the textbooks say to never argue with a dementia patient, although even without the illness you could never win an argument with Fiona, so we play along. Sometimes Mackenzie has to fetch her electric-blue Whistles coat – one of the very few items of clothing this once-stylish woman now insists on wearing, despite having a room full of outfits – and then Fiona and I leave the house as if I am taking her home. We walk around the block as she loudly proclaims, 'I'll never forgive you for tricking me,' and passers-by stare; then we are back home again, where she goes in and greets Mackenzie as if she hasn't seen him for days. She has forgotten about her mum and dad and is happy to sit down and eat another of her favourite Marks & Spencer Pink Lady apples.

After that, she will be visibly drained. Her brain is using up what small reserves of energy are left in her tiny frame. And then the house – or certainly her bedroom – is filled with the soundtrack of our current life. It never changes. Every day, several times a day, she'll say, 'Hey Google, play The Stylistics,' as she's transported back to her safe space, her teenage bedroom in Southampton. She begins to sing, word perfect and I stroke her hair as she says, 'Please don't leave me.'

Alzheimer's is the most awful disease, there is no way of sugar-coating it. The boys and I are being punished by it. But Fiona is the one having to live it every single day. And it's relentless, it just goes on and on. Fiona could outlive me. She could be here into her eighties, but she will never get any better and her quality of life will just go downhill. And there's absolutely nothing I can do to help her. All I can do is watch as the vast potential in this sparkling, vivacious woman is drained away from her. I can see the frustration in her eyes as it happens.

'Why have I had such bad luck?' she will ask me sometimes.

What can I say? It is just the worst luck.

And so, yes, writing this book has been very difficult for Fiona. Some memories from years ago remain, which she repeats over and over, but even those are becoming harder for her to find. The most recent events are the hardest for her to recall. Therefore, as the narrative of this book has progressed closer to the present day, it has become more difficult still – for both of us, in different ways.

Fiona was always authentically herself when she was on television and in her real life too. And that is what she would want now: to show that there is no Hollywood schmaltz with Alzheimer's. It's a difficult, painful disease and it's important people know that.

Some days, Fiona still likes to chat and answer the questions people ask her, but she is now unable to string together a story of events with the self-reflection and emotion you would normally find in an autobiography, so perhaps it is best to conclude this book in its final chapter in the 'Fiona way', by which I mean the 'authentic, honest' way, where you will read her words as they come to her now.

Sometimes those words and thoughts change from day to day. Sometimes they are contradictory. Sometimes they are laced with sadness. Sometimes Fiona puts on that mask of hopefulness she has so often worn. She is no longer the independent woman I fell in love with, but sometimes she is as stubborn as she has always been. Part of her is still the Fiona she told you about in the early chapters of this book, but much of her now is not.

I miss her. I miss my wife.

I'm afraid Fiona no longer remembers she is writing this book, so I will help prompt her for the next, final chapter to give you a snapshot of how she is doing. She will say she still likes to go out, but the truth is that it's a struggle to coax her out the house nowadays. And you'll pick up the little things she forgets. But this is her story and the last words should be from her. They may not all make perfect sense, but they are the real Fiona.

As for me? What do I really think? I think, *Fuck you, Alzheimer's!*

33

Fiona and Martin

———

March 2025

It is March 2025 and Fiona is sitting in the bright, airy kitchen of her home in south London, where she began this story.

Next to her sits Martin, who has just made them both a cup of tea. They drink and chat while Fiona tucks into a large slice of caramel shortbread.

Throughout the conversation, Martin has to prompt Fiona and remind her of events from recent weeks and months. She appears slimmer than ever and very fragile. Occasionally her eyes take on a vacant stare. Then Martin coaxes her back into the conversation by reminding her of a recent trip in the car and they chat about the shortbread and the television shows they watch together. A few moments later, it is all repeated.

Fiona still complains frequently of feeling internal physical pain – even though doctors are unable to identify exactly what may be the cause of this. Other times she seems to forget the pain entirely.

For a while, Fiona appears bright and bubbly – the way she always was. But clearly talking is tiring for her. The mental strain of trying to hide her confusion as the conversation goes on around her seems huge. Martin appears tired too. The patience he shows — helping his wife talk about her daily life and reminding her which tablets she needs to take or how to get to the bathroom in her own house — seems endless. But it must be exhausting.

And yet, as the couple scroll through old photographs on Martin's phone, there are moments when they laugh and retell family anecdotes with a warmth and affection that prove beyond doubt that, whatever this cruel disease may do, love is the greatest memory . . .

Martin: So, Fiona, it's a gorgeous spring day and the sun is finally shining. It's been a long winter, though, hasn't it? How are you feeling now?

Fiona: I'm OK. Yeah, I think I'm all OK.

M: And you're better than before Christmas?

F: Oh, I can't remember much of last year now. What was going on then?

M: Well, you were in a lot of pain.

F: Was I? What was that then?

M: Well, you were in terrible pain and we had to go to see a lot of consultants and finally one of them diagnosed the issue and he was able to operate on you.

F: Oh God, yes, that . . . Yes, that was horrible.

M: And I've left *This Morning* and I'm working on other projects so I've been around a bit more at home too.

F: Oh yes, you are around. Yes, that's nice.

M: But we don't go out so much, do we? You seem to prefer the security of your surroundings at home.

F: I do. Yes, I think so. But I wouldn't want to be at home all the time, though if I have to then I will.

M: You like being here, don't you?

F: I think so. It's funny but I can't remember a lot of what goes on – life just goes whoosh, doesn't it, and then that's it.

M: Does it bother you when you can't remember?

F: No.

M: And we still watch television together, don't we, and have a laugh? We watch *Dragons' Den* and *Dad's Army*.

F: Oh yes, *Dad's Army*. That's hilarious. And it's still going. I like things to laugh about. Life would be very odd if we didn't laugh at anything – or anyone!

M: And then I'll cook dinner. What do you like me to cook?

F: Oh, I don't know – I don't think about it really.

M: We look at some of the old pictures of Nat and Mackenzie when they were little. And they spend time with you whenever they can.

F: Yes, we see a lot of them so that's nice to have them around.

M: You were saying earlier that you missed your mum and you were asking where she's buried.

F: Yes, of course I think about my mum. Sometimes I think she is still here and then I remember that she isn't. That is so sad. And my dad.

M: But your brothers David and Andy both came around in the past week to visit.

F: Oh yes, we still stick together.

M: And your friend Amanda comes to see you and took you to get your hair coloured by her hairdresser.

F: Yes, she's a very good friend. We chat about husbands and all those things.

M: You're back on antidepressants, aren't you, Fiona, at the moment?

F: No, I'm not.

M: Yes, yes, you are – just a very mild dose just to cheer you up a bit.

F: When did that happen?

M: A couple of months ago – the doctors thought it might help you.

F: Oh.

M: Do you feel they are helping at all?

F: Not particularly, no – it all feels about the same. I don't like to talk about it, to be honest, because it's all pretty horrible. I just wish my mum was here – she was always laughing and joking. She was so sweet.

M: The publishers have announced that this book you are writing is due to come out this July, which is very exciting. There was a huge response to the news you had written a book. There were stories in the papers and they even discussed it on *Loose Women*.

F: Oh, I didn't know that. That's nice.

M: I think people feel it is inspiring that you are speaking about what you are dealing with and that it will be helpful for other people.

F: OK. Well, I think I have done all right with it although it doesn't stop me doing anything. But it is horrible.

M: Yes, although maybe you don't go out as much as you used to?

F: No. But I don't give it much thought . . . I knew it was there, but I don't even think about it now because if you do think about it, it's awful. Eurgh! I don't think about it because it has already done most of its horribleness. I don't give anything to Alzheimer's.

M: Sometimes you enjoy going to your room and you say to the smartspeaker: 'Hey Google, play The Stylistics' or 'Play Andy Williams'.

F: Oh yes, Andy Williams had such a warm voice. And I saw The Stylistics in concert before I even moved to London. I loved them – *'God bless you. You make me feel brand new.'* See, I can remember the words. That makes me happy.

M: Good . . . good.

F: It's just I would just rather *it* wasn't here. I pretend it's not here. I don't talk about it at all. It's awful it gets to some people and others are fine.

M: Yes, it's very cruel.

F: But I have . . . What was I going to say? Oh yes . . . I have what my mum would call 'a sunny disposition'.

M: Yes, Fiona. Yes, you do.

For More Information

The Alzheimer's Society: www.alzheimers.org.uk
Dementia Support Line: 0330 150 3456
Dementia UK: www.dementiauk.org
Alzheimer's Research UK: www.alzheimersresearchuk.org

There are dozens of questions we have asked ourselves and the experts over the past few years as we have dealt with the reality of Alzheimer's in our lives. We know many others going through the same ordeal will also be wondering about similar issues. So, here, Professor Catherine Mummery – who leads the cognitive disorders service at the National Hospital for Neurology at University College Hospital (where Fiona underwent her trial) and has been a senior investigator on more than twenty early-phase drug trials – will try to answer some of those questions.

We hope her insight, experience and honesty are of value to everyone reading this book.

Fiona: So I guess the first question is: why me? Why do some people get this terrible disease, particularly when we are still young, when other people can live to 100 and be untouched by it?

Professor
Mummery: Everybody asks this question at some point. The honest answer is that we have an idea of the risk factors of getting some form of dementia, such as Alzheimer's, but there is no exact formula as to who will get it and who will not. A very small percentage of cases are caused by a genetic change. One of the major factors is genetic – your apoE status – but this will increase your risk rather than cause Alzheimer's. However, for most people, it's a combination of factors that adds up to increase their chance of developing Alzheimer's at some point. If we lived long enough then most of us, at some point, would get Alzheimer's, because the biggest risk factor is age. The older you are, the more common it is. Other risk factors are your level of education, your vascular risk factors (raised blood pressure, diabetes, high cholesterol), whether you smoke, if you are suffering with isolation or mental health problems, if you have hearing diffi-culties . . . But, even if all of those things are fine, you still could get Alzheimer's disease. So the bottom line is it can be a case of bad luck.

F: So, if old age is the greatest risk factor, does that mean the disease is growing inside us for many years before we notice?

PM: Our bodies are all made up of proteins – in our brains, we have amyloid and tau proteins, which are critical to different brain functions. In someone who gets Alzheimer's disease, at some point the amyloid protein starts to misform and stops functioning normally. It becomes sticky, begins clumping together and gradually builds up. After a while, probably about twenty years, that starts to affect the tau protein, which then starts to spread from cell to cell and also begins clumping together. Between the two proteins, damage is caused to cells, which affects the brain. So, yes, this is a process that is going on for decades before someone even gets symptoms.

F: So could I have been diagnosed before I had symptoms? And would that have helped?

PM: At the moment, we have tests that can show evidence of these proteins misforming before someone has symptoms, but what they don't tell us is *when* someone is going to develop symptoms. So we don't use those tests to give a diagnosis. A diagnosis requires someone to have symptoms

313

and *then* we look for protein changes that confirm the diagnosis.

F: Wouldn't it be better to test everyone in their thirties so they can be prepared?

PM: Well, there is a big ongoing debate among researchers, because some of us do believe that we should make biological diagnoses upon seeing abnormal proteins, rather than waiting for symptoms. With new treatments coming through that may be able to slow the advance of symptoms, early detection will become even more important. If we waited to treat people with cancer only when they had symptoms, the survival rate would be far lower.

F: I was told that my Alzheimer's wasn't genetic but that I was predisposed to getting it – what does that mean?

PM: Less than 1 per cent of Alzheimer's is genetic, which is the term used when someone has a genetic mutation that produces amyloid in their brain and means they are almost 100 per cent certain to get the disease. That is often when they are still very young – in their thirties or forties. But those cases are extremely rare, only applying to around 20,000 people in the UK, out of about a million people with dementia. In other cases, when there has been a history of the disease in the family, there are genetic risk factors that won't guarantee someone will inherit the illness, but do mean they are predisposed to it or more likely to get it.

F: Do you think stressful periods in my life, such as waking up early to do *GMTV* while bringing up young children and caring for my parents, could have had an impact on what has happened?

PM: Often, if someone is in a very stressful situation, minor symptoms may start to show earlier than if they weren't stressed as the stress 'unmasks' the problem. But stress doesn't cause Alzheimer's to worsen. If you are tired and stressed then you have less reserve to cope with symptoms of *any* illness, including Alzheimer's.

Martin: Fiona and her mum both suffered with periods of depression during their lives. Could that have been a contributory factor for them? Or was it their Alzheimer's that caused their depression?

PM: Many people who get Alzheimer's disease do get depression. It is a depressing diagnosis. And, when people are diagnosed, there are often signs that they are already struggling with life. They're not showing any obvious Alzheimer's symptoms, but maybe they are overwhelmed at work or feeling anxious or in a low mood. And that can be a sign that the illness is coming, especially in young people with early-onset Alzheimer's. Those symptoms may be interpreted as depression or anxiety when really they are the beginnings of Alzheimer's. Social isolation as a result of depression can also be a risk factor in the likelihood of getting the disease, but neither is a direct cause.

M: What should a partner or family member do if they're concerned a loved one is suffering with memory loss?

PM: You have to take people very seriously and talk through their issues. It could well be stress, anxiety or exhaustion causing temporary memory loss, but it should not be ignored. We all know that when we are particularly stressed our memory can go to pot; we forget appointments or where we've put our car keys or glasses. But that is because we have diverted our attention away from thinking about those things and towards whatever it is we are stressed about. Forgetting what you had for breakfast that morning or how to get to the local shops is very different. If you are concerned that a loved one is struggling with that kind of memory loss, you should encourage them to make an appointment with a GP, who will be able to refer them for tests that can show whether there is something serious going on.

F: Is there anything, besides medication, that can be done to delay Alzheimer's advancing once symptoms have begun?

PM: Physical exercise helps – getting out of breath for thirty minutes three times a week is probably as good as any of the other medicines we have available right now. And mental exercise, which doesn't have to be brain games in a newspaper, but could be something like cooking a three-course dinner and serving it up on time. Or joining a club where you meet new, interesting people to chat with. Having a healthy diet is important too.

M: What's the best way for people to try to live after an Alzheimer's diagnosis?

PM: People have very different coping mechanisms. Some choose not to think about or discuss what is going on at all. I had one patient who referred to his Alzheimer's as Mr A. and would say: 'I'm not talking to Mr A. today, I'm ignoring him.' But other days he would want to deal with him and how he was feeling. I have other patients who swing between days of extreme despair and days when they have an amazing time doing something they love like watching sport. I tell my patients to 'play to your strengths' and do the things you enjoy, because much of your brain is still going to be working well for a long time. Your memory is a problem, but you can still walk for miles, see things well, paint, sing or do whatever it is that you love. It's about finding the things that enable you to see beyond the illness, for it to not become the centre of your life. If someone in a family had cancer, they wouldn't want every conversation to revolve around cancer – it is the same with Alzheimer's. And people with Alzheimer's should try to avoid things that frustrate them. Although it is difficult for my patients to accept that there are things they can no longer do, I remind them that taking a step back and getting help when needed can prevent them from feeling overwhelmed. Give yourself time and space. If having a conversation with more than one person is difficult, just explain that to people and they will understand.

M: Sometimes it feels as though Fiona is able to put on a great show for other people, but when she is at home alone with me she is far more withdrawn. Is that normal?

318

PM: Yes, that is very common. It is often the loved ones who feel the full force of the difficulties. But someone with Alzheimer's can feel exhausted a lot of the time. Talking to people and just managing life is like being in a mental gym. What was once automatic now involves a huge amount of effort. So, yes, when they get home, they are likely to be very tired. And there can also be changes in their behaviour. They might be as sweet as pie with someone they don't know, but then really unpleasant to their partner, lashing out verbally and physically. It is incredibly difficult and all I can say is try to get as much support as you can to give yourself a break. And make sure the person with Alzheimer's isn't getting overtired, which can make things worse. There are different things you can try to calm someone if they are agitated or distressed; it might be music or an activity they enjoy doing, such as painting or Sudoku, or a recording of a loved one's voice reassuring them – it varies. Sometimes there may also be particular carers who are able to calm the person in a way that their partner or child can't.

M: Do you think there will ever be treatments to cure Alzheimer's?

PM: It is an incredibly exciting time right now in terms of new treatments coming through for Alzheimer's – and for other dementias a little further down the line. There are drugs that have been approved for use in many countries that will slow the advance of symptoms for people in the very early stages of the disease. But this is just the beginning of what we will be able to achieve in future. Work is also ongoing on treatments that would stop misforming proteins from being produced in the first place, rather than just mopping them up. That may be a few years away, but it would be an incredible break-through. I think in the next twenty years we will reach a point where we will be able to manage Alzheimer's like a chronic disease – for example, how we have been able to manage HIV. People will still have it, but we will be able to diagnose it sooner – maybe through routine screening, as we do for breast cancer. And then we will be able to keep symptoms at a lower level or even prevent them from coming on at all. For people experiencing the impact of Alzheimer's right now, it remains incredibly difficult. But I do believe there are treatments to feel very hopeful about on the horizon.